Coming out

By Jean Murphy

ISBN: 1-905451-24-5

A CIP catalogue for this book is available from the National Library.

All names contained in this story have been changed to protect the identity of persons mentioned.

This book was published in cooperation with
Choice Publishing & Book Services Ltd, Ireland
Tel: 041 9841551 Email: info@choicepublishing.ie
www.choicepublishing.ie

Preface

I was born in 1946 and was one of a family of eight children. I lived in a remote part of north County Dublin, and left school and home at seventeen to work in Dublin city. From the age of eleven I corresponded with a pen-pal in Connecticut. Creative writing became a favoured hobby of mine.

I am married to Ciaran Murphy, and we have three grown children, Nicola, Robert and Declan. A very special addition to the family is Mia, daughter to Nicola and her husband Aadil.

At the age of fifty-three I suffered an acute stroke, leaving me completely paralyzed on the left side of my body. I became a wheelchair user, and was prompted to write an account of what happened to bring this about. I was so disappointed at not being able to return to the work-place after rearing my children that I wanted to produce a piece of work of my own. That also prompted me to write this book, Coming Out. I hope that this book helps in some small way to encourage other stroke patients, and other people who become disabled.

CHAPTER ONE

The Early Days

I met Billy Heaney to-day. It brought back memories - some happy and some very painful.

"Hi Billy," I called out. He looked at me, but he didn't recognise me at all. I removed my sunglasses. His hand slowly went up to his mouth.

"I'm Jean Murphy, Ciaran's wife," I said by way of re-introduction.

'Ah, Now I remember. Ah yeah. Ciaran and the dog. Cindy wasn't it?' He still looked perplexed.

'It's Jessy now Billy. Cindy has gone to doggy Heaven. The last time I met you was in the Botanic Gardens, Billy. You were with your wife, and Ciaran was pushing me in a wheelchair.'

'Now I remember. How are you keeping anyway?'

'I'm grand thanks Billy. Sure as long as I can get out and about I'm fine.' We said our good-byes, and I headed into the post office. Someone held the door open for me, to let me through, and I joined the queue for stamps. Again, when I was leaving a woman opened the door, and I thanked her. It brings a great smile to my face when people are so kind and helpful.

My journey home took me to the busy main road, and on to the traffic lights on Ballymun Road. When I got the green man I pointed my joystick forward, and off I drove, first glancing to see that the traffic had come to a standstill. I came up through Hamstead Park. Along the way I met several acquaintances out walking their dogs.

As I drove along through the quiet park my mind wandered back to the weekend prior to my stroke, when I sat down to Sunday dinner with my husband Ciaran and children. Declan, always being the comic in the family talking his way through Sunday dinner, and Robert, two years older than Declan, sitting quietly eating everything in front of him. And Nicola, my only daughter, rushing through the front door at the last minute, having driven over from her flat in Rathmines to spend a little time with us, and to take a break from her studies. It all seemed such a long time ago. Then, I could get up from the table, and cater to my family, using both of my hands.

It's five years on since that awful morning in January when my life changed drastically.

CHAPTER TWO

The Early days

My head was exploding with pain. I went back to bed after making breakfast for Ciaran. The doctor had visited me the day before at my request. He had checked my blood pressure; it was high again at one-hundred and eighty over one hundred. I told him about the pins and needles in my left foot and leg. I felt full of influenza or something.

Declan was not too far away, so I phoned him and asked him if he could come home and help me with some housework. It was a relief when he came home promptly. I went back to sleep relieved that somebody was near.

At eleven o'clock I decided to get up and do some housework. I tried to move, but I couldn't. For a moment I thought I had slept on my left arm. I reached my right hand over to lift the sleeping left one. As my right hand touched my breast there was no feeling there. Then I knew something was seriously wrong. There was no sensation. I reached down to feel my leg; there was no sensation there either. My hand went up to my face. There was no sensation in my neck. I reached to the floor for my slipper, wondering how I was going to tell Declan that I thought I had had a stroke. I banged on the floor. I didn't want to scare him.

'Mam I haven't got the music on loud' Declan called up the stairs.

'Declan, could you come up please?' I asked him calmly. 'I think I've had a stroke or something. Could you ring for an ambulance?' I asked him, explaining that I had lost sensation in all of my left side. I tried to hide my worry. I wanted to shield Declan from this awful situation.

'Hello, could you send an ambulance out to my mother. She's all messed up on one side of her body. Right thanks.' I heard him say into the phone. I was too tired to care about anything. I asked Declan to put my dressing gown into a bag, also my slippers.

We waited for what-seemed-like twenty minutes. 'Please ring again Declan.' I asked Declan. This time I called into the phone for them to please come to my aid. Very quickly I could hear the sound of the ambulance coming up Ballymun Road. I knew it was for me, and now the thoughts of being taken off to hospital really frightened me.

The ambulance crew arrived up the stairs. One of them felt my foot, 'Can you feel that?'

'No,' I replied. I could feel no sensation as he touched my left hand or leg either. They got me out of bed, and put me in a chair to carry me to the waiting ambulance. They took me down the stairs on a stretcher. Declan came in the ambulance with me. An oxigen mask was put over my nose. I remember nothing more for about two days after that moment.

'We are sending your scans to Beaumont Hospital to be studied by the neuro-surgeons,' a doctor said close to my ear. My hand went up to my head to where the terrible pain was. 'We want to find out what caused your stroke.' He said.

'Could you describe the pain?' Another doctor asked me.

'It feels as if I had been hit by an iron bar right across the side of my head.' I answered the doctor. A nurse told me not to keep my hand up to my head or it would make my arm ache. I have vague recollections of Ciaran, my husband, being present. Sometimes only Nicola was there. She was a great comfort to me. She didn't sound frightened, so I thought there must not be very much wrong. I would probably be better in a few days. It was probably only a mild stroke, like the ones my Mother had, and she recovered fairly well after them.

A nurse checked my blood pressure regularly. When she asked which arm was my bad arm I promptly told her that that was not a bad arm. I told my hand that it was a good hand. 'Mam, they'll think you've lost your marbles if you keep on talking to your hand like that.' Nicola was a little embarrassed when I talked to my hand, but it seemed the most natural thing for me to do. I felt really sorry for my arm and hand, and especially when the nurses called it a bad hand, or a bad arm. We agreed that we would refer to my left hand or arm or leg as weak rather than bad. I talked to my hand and re-assured it that it was a good hand, and that it had worked for me for fifty-three years. Nicola looked bemused at me.

Pillows were placed under my head, and my left hand was splayed across a pillow. I constantly asked for a bedpan. When I couldn't pass water the nurse told me that they would insert a catheter into my bladder. It sounded horrific, but in fact I don't remember anything other than a cold sensation in that area. I continued to look for a bedpan, so the nurse lifted the bag for urine collection and showed it to me. After that I had no more need for a bedpan. I remember being settled in a new bed upstairs.

Time passed in a strange sort of way. I didn't know if it was night or day. I was uncomfortable in every way. I looked for a sick dish, but then I would not be able to get sick.

The speech therapist came along to check my throat and speech. She spoon-fed yogurt to me, and checked as I swallowed. She made a chart of instructions, and put it on the wall behind my bed. Food was to be chopped up small, and I was to be discouraged from talking while eating. I felt like a baby.

Family came to visit at night. Jo, my sister-in-law, put her arms around me. I thought it was the end; I could hardly breathe, and I was too exhausted to explain. My brother, Martin and his wife Angela were there, somewhere close to my bed.

'Come on Marti, ' Angela said to my brother, 'she's not able for visitors.' It was a relief when all the visitors left the ward. That was one of my worst nights. The Hospital Chaplain came to see me. She was a large woman with a very kindly face. She seemed to understand my distress. She stood beside my bed for a while. It was reassuring to have someone close to me. I was very distressed.

'This poor lady is over-whelmed.' She told the nurse. The nurse pulled the curtain around a little so that it was quiet for me.

Holly came on duty at eight o'clock. She was like an Angel sent specially to help. There was noise coming from somewhere close-by. It sounded like footsteps hurrying anxiously.

'Nurse I'm really frightened' I told Holly. 'Will you stay with me for a little while?' Holly sat with me. 'Holly, I keep on hearing noises, and it's really frightening,' she fixed my pillows, and talked about what had happened to me. Holly explained that the Intensive Care ward was near and that family would be visiting when some member was very ill. I said a prayer in my mind for all the patients who were in Intensive Care.

She then showed me a beautiful blue dressing gown which Rita, my sister-in-law had brought to me, and she folded it and put it into my locker. She showed me lovely body lotions which were brought to me by family members, and put them away in my drawer. It was a relief when the nurses arrived with the drugs trolly and they gave us our medicines. The lights were lowered, and we tried to settle down to sleep.

Holly was still around, and she gave me the bell just in case I was worried. I felt her woolly cardigan between my fingers. 'Holly you are like a woolly lamb,' I told her. I wanted to put my arms around her to feel safe. I felt like a tiny child, vulnerable and small.

'I'll just be over here settling down the other patients for the night,' Holly assured me.

'I love you Holly,' I told her, and I settled down to sleep.

After breakfast next morning the dietician came and she made out a chart indicating to the staff that I ate a gluten-free diet. All cereals were out; also any food containing wheat, oats barley and rye, were to be excluded from my diet. She pinned the chart of instructions behind my bed.

The patient across from me brought over a prayer and handed it to me.

When the day nurses came on duty they immediately started work on baths and showers or basin washes. I couldn't move without help, and the thought of being dunked in a bath seemed like a nightmare. When they came to wash me they told me that they were going to put me sitting out after a wash. I had confidence in the big tall sister. I knew she wouldn't let me fall. After a basin wash and a change of clothes they put on my new silky dressing gown, and they helped me across to the leather buxton chair. They immediately went to work making the bed and putting on fresh sheets. Suddenly I went flying down the leather buxton chair, and went sliding across the floor on my bottom, and landed across the room with my feet under a tall table of medical bits and pieces.

The nurses calmly helped me back into the chair, and the silky dressing gown was put away until I was better. A doctor was sent for to check that no damage had been done. My big toe constantly pained and a blood test was done to check for gout. I made up my mind there and then that I wouldn't complain so quickly again as blood tests were ordered if you as much as sneezed.

I was petrified that they would dunk me into a big bath of water. 'I hope they don't put me into the gas chamber,' I made a joke with Ciaran. I thought, somehow, that he understood me, but he didn't. After all he was looking at a very sick person, and it transpired that he didn't understand that I was joking. He knew about my dislike of water. It was all so strange being in a world of my own with nobody understanding. I felt isolated in some way.

Next morning nurse Celine was bathing me. 'Why did you tell your husband that we were going to put you into a gas chamber?' she scolded me. 'I can't nurse you if you're going to be depressed like this all the time, Jean.'

'I'm not depressed nurse,' I told her back. 'I don't like water that's all, and I was making a joke with Ciaran and I thought he understood me, you see.'

A large bouquet of flowers arrived for me from my Aunt in Australia, and Celine looked about the ward for a vase, obviously bothered at having to do so. 'Just yank them under the bed for the moment.' I said to her.

'Please and thank you would be nice, Jean,' she corrected me.

'Please and thank you nurse.' I said there and then.

Eithne, one of my girl friends, came to visit. She was carrying a basket of beautiful flowering polyanthus. 'How are you Jean?' I couldn't believe what happened when Ciaran phoned.'

'I'm o.k., sort of o.k. I don't know how I am, bloody awful I suppose is how I am.'

'At least you didn't lose your speech,' Eithne tried to console me.

'I lost enough so I did.' I said wearily.

'Well you're still Jean anyway.' Eithne declared.

'I love you, Eithne,' I was too tired for any more conversation. Eithne sat with me for awhile. She read the notices put on the wall behind my bed.

'And what can you eat, Jean if you can't eat all those things?' Eithne enquired studying the chart.

'I can eat all kinds of meat and fruit and vegetables and I make my own bread at home, so I don't go hungry.'

'Poor Ciaran, his eyes looked red from crying. It must have been a terrible shock for him.' Eithne said. She kissed me good-bye, and left me to sleep for a while.

Next my friend Anne arrived with a basket of beautiful yellow flowers arranged very attractively. 'I won those at the I.C.A. last night.' She said. Before too long another friend, Phil came in carrying another basket of lovely pink and purple flowers. Flowers adorned the window across from me. On my locker were flowers brought from friends and family. I just wanted to vanish into sleep.

'We will be true to thee till death. Oh, how our hearts beat high with joy, when 'ere we hear that glorious word. Faith of our Father's Holy Faith. We will be true to thee till death.' Next morning I woke myself up singing that Hymn. I sang out loud and clear.

'There's no singing allowed on the ward, Jean.' nurse told me. I woke singing at the top of my voice. In fact I woke everyone else up as well. It was only about six o'clock in the morning.

'Sorry nurse, I didn't know I was singing.' I apologised. 'I can't sing anyway nurse.'

I made up my mind that to-day I would try harder. I didn't want to be in any more trouble.

After being washed and freshened up for the day the nurse told me they were sending the porter to collect me to go to the gym. 'I don't want to go nurse,' I pleaded. 'I can't walk, and they'll make me try walking, and I might fall.' A few minutes passed and the porter was up and waiting. The nurses got me up, and off I was wheeled, down to the elevator. We travelled along the link to the new wing, the porter saying 'good morning' to his colleagues as he pushed me along. The fresh air felt good as we passed through the lobby area.

The physiotherapist pointed the porter in the direction of the hoist where I waited a moment for attention. I looked around a huge place with patients being helped out of wheelchairs and onto bench beds. Some patients had only half legs. I felt slightly sick at the thought of what might have happened to them. Next my turn came. I didn't know what to expect. The therapist introduced herself to me. Her name was Ursula. I liked her straight away. She explained as she put the hoist around and under me that they were going to lever me over to the bench bed to work on my weak limbs. I was very frightened of falling all the time and it was a relief when I was finally winched and released. Two physiotherapists worked on my left leg and arm. They then tried to get me into a sitting position. I kept falling down to the left side, but they got me back up sitting again. They had amazing patience. I had to practise going from side to side to strengthen the muscles in the left side of my bum. Bum is the hospital word for bottom I soon discovered.

'Don't let me fall,' I called out as they winched me back over to the wheelchair. The brakes were released, and off I was wheeled back along the link. The porter just lifted me back onto the chair beside my hospital bed.

'Now young one, that wasn't too bad was it? 'The porter ventured a joke.

'How did physiotherapy go?' nurse Maureen asked when I got back.

'It was exhausting.' I told her as she chopped my dinner into small pieces. I tried to eat a little bit of food after all the hard work. Nurse Maureen helped me into bed for a rest before I was sent for a brain scan later on in the afternoon. I slept for a little while.

The porter arrived calling out my name. He was pushing the big leather buxton chair for me to go to the xray department. I could hardly stay awake as they lifted me from the bed, and back into the buxton chair, and off we went again down through the lift, and along the link. And then we were there. The porter parked me beside other weary-looking patients, waiting their turn to be scanned. I wished I could walk and get up and run away, but I couldn't. I had to sit there with patients looking at each other for signs of sickness. An old woman kept staring at me. I was conscious that my face was crooked. Nicola had shown it to me in the mirror.

'Why are you staring at me?' I asked her. She looked away. I checked again. No she was not looking That was a relief, but I felt guilty in case I had hurt her feelings. It seemed that my speech was on automatic pilot. I didn't want anyone looking at my crooked face.

Nicola arrived to visit in the evening.

'Hi. How are we to-day? I believe you had another brain scan.'

'I had one done to-day, but I don't know if I had another one done.'

'Do you remember when you came in? Well you had one done the next day. Then you were sent up here to Saint Cecelia's ward. I'm going to give you a little diary, and we'll write things down, so you will be able to remember things like who came to visit you, and so on. D'ont worry, Mam, until you feel better.'

Nicola found a small diary in her hand-bag, and she started writing at the twenty-fifth of January. 'You'll want to be able to thank people for flowers and presents when you're well again.' She said, as she wrote for me. 'And who was in this afternoon can you remember?' And the diary was started. 'Do you remember who came to see you in casualty?'

'No, I can't remember.'

'The nurses were really nice in casualty. When they asked you questions, you were able to answer. It's strange that you can't remember.' Nicola chatted to me.'And the male nurse bringing you the bedpan, can you remember that?' She was teasing me.

'I remember once asking for a bedpan and when the nurse didn't come with one I just wet the bed, because I thought my bladder might burst like a baloon, and she asked me if I had lost control of my bladder, and I told her that when they didn't come with the bedpan that I decided to wet the bed. I don't think she was amused. I'm too tired to talk any longer Nicola. Do you mind if I go asleep?'

Next morning the doctor was around bright and early. 'We're moving you to a different ward to-day Jean,' she told me ' We are very pleased with your progress. You are doing very well.'

'I don't want to move doctor,' I protested. 'I like it here.'

'You will like the other ward too. The patients there are not as sick as they are here. You'll settle in there too.' Two nurses came promptly to pack me up and pack me off. They had two plastic bags. My clothes were put into the larger one.

'Don't forget her slippers,' one nurse reminded the other one. Next the little bag was open for the things in my drawer.

'What's in this?' asked the other nurse.

'It's just rubbish, here put it in this,' she said as she quickly picked up my face creams, my precious mirrors for looking at my crooked face, hand creams, reading glasses, and all other bits and pieces which my family had brought into hospital for my needs, were chucked into a plastic bag, for my next stop.

'I don't want to go,' I pleaded with the busy nurses. The porter arrived, and a few minutes later we were on our way down the lift and into the new ward; the bags loaded up on the buxton chair beside me, and baskets of flowers piled on any bit of space available. I looked around. The ward had six beds, all occupied by elderly-looking patients. He deposited me beside a freshly-made bed, and handed my file to the nurse.

Sister came over to talk to me. 'I'm not going to like it here. I didn't want to move.' I said to Sister.

'This is like all the other wards in the hospital. You'll settle in soon. I'll be back in a minute.' And off Sister went to get a form to fill in details of what things I had with me.

CHAPTER THREE

The Early Days

In the bed opposite a grey-haired old lady sat staring at me. Her eyes were fierce-looking, and her hair hung shoulder-length. She watched me carefully. I felt frightened of her in case she might walk over to me and touch me. I could hardly move to defend myself. Her nails were long, and claw-like, and her nose was long, giving her a look of Ron Moody from the film Oliver. Beside her was a lovely old lady just sitting leisurely watching the world go by.

'Ah God help her all the same. Isn't she very young?' The old woman said loudly to the lovely old lady beside her. I wished she hadn't taken an interest in me at all. She kept staring at me, her eyes focussed on me alone. A young nurse came along to her.

'Now Masie we'll do your hair for you,' and she set about combing the old woman's hair, and putting it tied back behind her head.

'They don't care what they send down to us down here,' Masie said looking at me with a weary fed-up look on her face.

'I told you not to be passing remarks at other people,' the lovely old lady said to Masie. She looked away at last. When the nurse finished doing her hair she wanted to go to the toilet.

'Where's the bucket. I want to do me pee?' she asked of the other old lady-Kitty.

'Here come on and I'll take you to the bathroom.' Kitty said. The two old women made their way out together helping each other along as they went. They made a sad-looking picture, stooped over as they went along.

Beside me was Kara, a lovely young woman of about twenty-eight. I was glad to see one young face in the ward. She said 'hello' and asked me how was I feeling. I felt more settled then, and the nurse told me I probably wouldn't be moved again. This morning I was scheduled to have a glucose-tolerance test. It involved having a blood test, followed by a large drink of sweet orange. Some time later another blood test was taken.

Masie was back on watch, her eyes searching out anything out of the ordinary. Once in my new bed, I was able to pull the sheet over my nose so that I didn't have to worry about her. Kitty sat serenely in her chair keeping Masie under control. I tried to rest before visiting time.

Visiting time brought children, grandchildren, and great grandchildren to visit Masie. It was like a picnic with mothers handing out packets of crisps to the children sitting on her bed. 'Be quiet now or the doctor will come with a big needle,' one of the mothers told her child. The child was so busy stuffing crisps into his mouth, washed down with lemonade, that he didn't even hear what she said. It was a great relief when a nurse announced that visiting time was over.

The Physiotherapist came up to me and planned my visits to the gym. The porter would collect me at nine a.m. and take me to the gym, and he would take me back at eleven. After lunch I would be taken back for a short while for more physiotherapy.

The first night was very worrying in my new ward. When the drugs trolley came round the nurses offered Masie her 'vitamins' but she refused to take any, telling them that she never took a tablet in her life and she wasn't going to start taking tablets now. 'They are good for you Masie,' the staff nurse said to her. She wasn't having any of it. Before long we all had our medication, except Masie, and we were in our beds settling down for the night. The nurse gave me the bell in case I needed to ask for a bedpan during the night. I was glad to have it in case the old lady came over to me. The thought of her long nails was just terrifying. I missed Holly, and wished she was there to comfort me now.

Suddenly Kara let out a scream which alerted all the night nurses. They came rushing in from next-door. It was Masie out of her bed. She had come over to Kara and put her hands on Kara's feet. Now Kara was laughing, calling out

'Masie you nearly gave me a heart attack.'

Masie was ordered back to her bed. Again she was offered her 'vitamins' but she refused them once more. She was well tucked in for the night, and the rest of us sick patients settled down to sleep.

'There are three cows outside the winda.' Masie shouted. 'Isn't that terrible having cows outside the windas. What would anyone think? You ought to be ashamed having cows in the front garden.' Kara started to laugh out loud. Other patients complained, and said that Masie should be sent to a private room for the night. The nurses said that they wished there was a room for her, but unfortunately there wasn't. I wondered if we were going to be kept awake all night. The lights were lowered again. I was exhausted and sick. I needed to sleep. Kara told me that Masie had alzheimers disease.

'Go to sleep Masie, and give us all a break.' Kara whispered across the room. All was quiet when a young man came into our room. I rang the bell, thinking it was a patient from the men's ward. The nurses came in quietly telling us that John was a male nurse, and that he was going to help take Masie out of the ward for the night. He got a buxton chair, and soon the noisy old lady was taken off all wrapped up cosily and taken out so the rest of us patients could get some rest. I imagined her having a glass of wine and lounging in a beautiful room with a television set. I went to sleep thinking happy thoughts.

February mornings were still dark when we woke in our hospital ward. In the quiet of the ward there was time to think of one's situation, but not for very long. 'Porridge or boiled egg?' Delia called out as she lifted up the trays for breakfast. The nurse came along to help me up into a sitting position. She pulled out the back rest and placed pillows behind me. I asked for a boiled egg. Delia cut the top off for me, and I tried to eat it as best I could with one hand. 'Anyone for a second cup?' asked Delia in a motherly fashion. I loved a second cup of tea in the morning. I began to feel comforted at last.

At eight o'clock the day nurses came on duty, fresh from their beds and off the tired night staff went until night-time again.

Masie was wheeled back into the ward comatose with sleep. 'Here's your porrige, ' Delia said loudly trying to arouse Masie. Delia went on to the men's ward adjoining ours, wheeling the breakfast trolly in front of her. The ward was quiet after breakfast, and we patients kept quiet knowing that we wanted to keep her ladyship asleep a bit longer.

Staff nurse Maureen came to me and encouraged me to wash my hair. 'How can I wash my hair lying on my back in bed?' I asked her. She had a way. She went off and fetched a flat basin suitable for placing at the back of the bed and it was possible, that way, to wash and rinse hair. I called her Mr. Motivator, as she could encourage patients to do anything. She blow-dried my hair as well. I looked a mess, but I smelled better.

Phil, one of the porters, collected me for physiotherapy. 'The speech-therapist wants to see you first, Jean,' Phil told me. I enjoyed the feel of fresh air as we approached the lobby. The speech therapist showed me a range of exercises to do daily in order to strengthen my facial muscles, and to help stop me from dribbling on the weak side of my face. 'A. E. I .O.U.' I said out loud. She gave me a chart of exercises to take back to the ward to practise during the weekend when there was plenty of free time.

Phil was called to take me on to Ursula the physiotherapist. We worked hard on bum exercises in order to get me sitting up properly in the wheelchair. I kept falling over to the weak side. I had to try to remember to sit up straight. It was all very tiring, but I started to feel a little better. Ursula praised me for trying so hard. She encouraged me to sit out of bed when I was taken back to the ward. After twelve o'clock lunch, the drugs trolley came round. Anything for the bowels Kara?' Staff nurse asked Kara as she went along.

'Gun powder,' Kara replied in a strong Cavan accent, laughing in her lovely pleasant way. I asked the nurses to help me get back into bed for a short nap before my next trip down to the gymnasium. Visiting time was in full swing when I got back from therapy. I was exhausted. Nurse's aid, Irene helped me back into bed to rest for a while before tea time.

When someone came to visit me at this time in the afternoon I was very often asleep after such a busy time exercising. Many times I woke to find some of my family sitting by my bedside while I slept. And many times I woke to find flowers left by somebody who had come to visit, but who didn't like to wake me. My illness sent shock waves through my family.

CHAPTER FOUR

Settling in

Saturday morning was quiet in the ward. The Hospital Chaplain came round with Communion to us patients before breakfast. Therapy stopped for the weekend, giving patients a welcome break and a rest. Karen, the other nurses aid in the ward came over to see if I wanted a shower or a basin wash. Now that there was plenty of time I agreed to a shower, hoping that she would be able to get me from the bed to the buxton chair, and then into the shower without letting me fall. Karen was a tiny girl, and she looked about sixteen years old, but she told me she was twenty-four. She assured me that she would be able. 'Sure you're like a little bird, Jean.' Karen said to me. She got me safely out of bed and off we went to the bathroom. There was a variety of washing facilities there.

'Close the windows please, Karen.' I asked as she helped me off with my clothes. The place had just been cleaned by Noreen, and it was cold with all the windows open. Getting me onto the shower seat was difficult, but Karen was confident, and she immediately inspired confidence in me. It felt good to be clean and fresh all over. Karen went out and got cream for my dry skin. She put fresh clothes on me, and brought me back to the ward. She put me sitting out in the big buxton chair. The buxton chair felt comfortable to sit in, but it sounded awful when it was being pushed along. It sounded like an old rusty wheelbarrow. It's arms were bandaged heavily, making it look as if it had been in a serious accident.

At ten-thirty a cup of tea was served, or soup for patients who wanted that. Masie was just waking up from her long sleep down the corridor. I wasn't afraid of her any longer. Most of the time she was in bed, and she slept a lot more as the days went on.

Kara was going home. The doctor had just given her the good news, but she would be back in a few weeks. She was having complications with her diabetes. I gave her some make-up, which Nicola had brought into me. 'I'm going to miss you Kara.' I told her, and I wondered who I might have next, close to my bed.

'You'll get better Jean. My mum had a stroke, and one day her arm shot up in the air and started working again. Keep doing the exercises. Your face is better already.' I was so glad to see the improvement in the shape of my face. I took out my chart of speech exercises and began.

'A, E, I, O, U.' Kara had her shower, and she arrived back in the ward with a big bunch of daffodils for me. She had made her way down to the florist in the lobby of the hospital to get them. Soon her partner collected her and we hugged each other goodbye. Her bed was immediately stripped down and washed and prepared for the next patient.

After visiting time a tiny lady was wheeled into the ward, and she was helped into Kara's bed beside me. She had soft grey hair, lightly permed, with a hint of a blue rinse through it. Her family left, and the doctor came along to see her. Masie was alert to her every move. 'Ah, God help her all the same.'

Kitty told her to stop passing remarks at people. The doctor went next to see Kitty. She was to be released next week to a nursing home. I wondered why, as she was quite a fresh looking lady. Next, he went to look at Masie. 'I never took a tablet in me life doctor.' she told him. He then spoke to her daughter. She was being released in a few days to be looked after by her daughter at home. Masie continued to comment on the little lady, 'Ah, God help her, she'll soon be on her way.' Her daughter was embarrassed.

'Sherrup Mammy, or you'll be trun out,' she said giving her mother a harsh look. She handed her a fresh bag of crisps and tried to engage her in conversation to divert her attention from the new patient. I was relieved that Masie had lost interest in me. The ward was quiet except for the sound of crisps being munched.

'Is SHE not dead yet?' Masie said aloud looking over, remembering the old lady with the blue rinse.

'Im owa here Mammy, enoughs enough.' and off the

daughter stormed, picking up her bags as she went. I wondered how on earth they were going to be able to look after her at home. Soon word got out that Masie was going home on Wednesday next. At last, we were going to be able to relax and recover our health.

Sunday morning was quiet with the television on over the door, for those of us who were interested in the prayer service. I listened to the words, contemplating them. 'Jesus left the boat and walked on the water to where the disciples were standing. The boat was tossed by the waves and wind, and went into the sea. When the disciples saw Jesus they were afraid, and they thought it was a spirit. Jesus told them to be of good cheer, and not to be afraid. Peter walked on the water to go to Jesus, but he felt afraid and began to sink. Jesus told them to have faith, and that they could do many things. If they were in fear they would fall.' For me this message was very important. I was afraid of falling in physiotherapy. I was afraid of being dunked into a bath of water and I was afraid of Masie. And so far none of my fears had come to fruition. Now, I must go forward without fear.

'A, E, I, O, U. Um, go, to, do.' I got on with my speech exercises to try to correct my sagging face muscles.

Ciaran arrived in early to visit me. It was only eleven o' clock in the morning. 'You look brighter today Jean,' he said, looking relieved. 'You've been through the mill.'

'You must have been up early,' I said, 'have you been out with Jessie in the park?' I asked Ciaran, barely able to think of Jessie, our lovely furry dog, without my lip quivering. We chatted about the lads and Nicola. They had all been through a terrible shock at my illness. I felt guilty being so wrapped up in myself, but it had been a terrible period of suffering, those first few days and first weeks for me, and as much as I could do was to get by, hour by hour, or from one day to the next. At last I felt the worst was over.

CHAPTER FIVE

Getting Stronger

It was a bright Monday morning, and I woke early to see a rich, pale blue sky. Little white fluffy clouds raced across it one after another, like young lambs playing chasing in a field. On my window-sill was a beautiful vase of daffodils sent in by Marie, my neighbour. Suddenly, and surprisingly, a magpie swooped down and took a beakfull of twigs from a flat roof, and busily flew off again. Nature was working well in the outside world; the birds were building their nests, and the ground was producing flowers to brighten our lives after the long Winter. There was good reason to be happy. I was beginning to feel stronger, although I had some really bad days when I thought I was going to crack. The bad patches passed when I slept off the feelings of exhaustion.

Delia wheeled in the breakfast trolley. 'Good morning girls. Who's for porrige, boiled egg or flakes?' I began to enjoy food at last. My sense of taste was improving. Delia helped me remove the top of the egg, and I ate it using one hand to poke up bits.

The night nurses helped patients up into a sitting position, pulling out back rests, before going off night duty. They were going to the hospital restaurant for a 'big fry-up' before heading off for a week's break after doing a week of nights. We wished them a good time on their break, and looked forward to seeing them back again on day duty. We patients in hospital held our nurses in high esteem.They worked long hours, and never complained.

The doctors were already in the men's ward on their rounds. We were next for visitation. Soon it was my turn. 'You are doing very well Jean,' Dr Lawlor told me. 'We have the results from your scans, and you are doing well in physio. Your stroke was caused by high blood pressure. You had a heavy bleed in the right side of your head causing your left side to become paralyzed.' She then examined my leg, testing for sensation, and also my arm. So far there was no sensation, but I was improving in other ways. I was not feeling as exhausted as I had been in the beginning. 'We have asked the doctor from the Rehabilitation Centre in Dun Laoghaire to call in to see you, Jean.' And then they were on their way to another ward. I wondered if I might be sent out to Dun Laoghaire to the Rehabilitation Center.

The haemothologist arrived with her cart full of needles and tubes for taking blood. I pulled the sheet up over my head in the hope that I would be forgotton, but there was no way out when Emma had your name in the computer. A notice on her cart read 'Heart your Haemotologist.' Emma was a very pleasant young woman, and she got to know us patients, and knew how to get the best out of us. In the beginning I refused to give blood samples when I was very ill.

Noreen arrived next with her polishers and shiners. Noreen's laughter could be heard long before she came into the ward. 'Mornin girls.'

'Mornin Noreen,' we called out. Showers and basin washes were in full swing, and as soon as we were out of our beds fresh linen was put on, and the day nurses were working hard. By nine a.m. I was washed, dressed, fed and sitting in the buxton chair ready for collection.

'You're looking very well this morning Jean,' Phil complimented me as we set off for the gymnasium. I liked going out of the ward now every morning. Phil told me about what was happening in the city, and we chatted as we went along the link. Other patients were being brought to the therapies, and soon we got to know each other, and greeted one another as we went on our way.

I was put standing with a large support by my right side. I had to reach to the left for a ring and put it on the ring board to the right side.Ursula worked hard with me, pushing the ring boards further away, and insisting that it was important that I work hard in these early weeks. It was more like a game for me, leaving the ring number thirteen until last, and hoping that I wouldn't fall. Somehow it escaped my mind that in fact they were trying to get me up and going on my feet. My brain was incapable of understanding very much in these early weeks. I laughed when I dropped a ring, as if it was a game. Next she got the bean bags. I had to reach over to take a bag from one bucket and reach over to put it across into the other bucket.

The Occupational Therapist dropped in to see how I was getting on in physiotherapy, and she gave me an appointment to go to her department in the afternoon.

Mark wheeled me back to the ward. My friend Grainne was waiting there for a short visit. She had her granddaughter with her in the buggy. 'I just dropped in for a quick visit, is it alright would you say, Jean?' Grainne whispered as she sat down in my corner. We had a grand chat and Grainne brought me a bundle of shiny magazines. I waved them goodbye, and dinner arrived with Delia treating us like her very own children.

'Now eat every bit of that chicken. It will do you good.' She said to me. And she always came back with a lovely cup of tea. After lunch I had an audience of nurses looking through the shiny magazines

'I'll be back later for a chat.' Karen promised as she went down to help for a while in accident and emergency department.

'You have your lippo on to-day, Jeannie,' nurse Gillian remarked. I was glad to see Gillian back on day duty after her break in the country. She seemed to transmit her boundless energy to the patients. Her dimples and her shiny black pony tail caught your eye as she passed in and out of the ward. She was jovial with the patients too.

'Had you a nice time on your week off Gillian?' I asked her.

'Yeah, it was great Jeannie.' And off she was gone to the next bed checking the blood pressures, and temperatures of each patient. She looked like someone in love. She had a mischieveous look in her very gait of going.

'Must be something good in Cork?' I teased her when she came back.

'Wouldn't you love to know Jeannie.'

CHAPTER SIX

Occupational Therapy

Mark came at two o'clock to collect me for Occupational Therapy. He brought up a normal-looking wheelchair. 'I want to go in one of these wheelchairs in future, Mark. I prefer this type of wheelchair. I don't like those buxton chairs, and especially not the one with the arms bandaged. It looks like an accident case. And now it's called 'Jean's buxton' if you wouldn't mind.'

'Come on young one' Mark said in his usual teasing way. He helped me from the armchair, beside my bed, into the wheelchair.

'What age are you, Mark?' I asked him

'Forty-one,' came the reply as we wheeled off out down to the elevator.

'I'm fifty-three. That means I'm no young one, Mark.' I said, wanting to think I was like a young one.

'Well you look like a young one to me.' Mark laughed, as we went along. Mark helped no end to repair my crushed ego. When I looked at my left hand I told myself that I still looked like a young one. I wondered what the therapist was going to do with me. I supposed she was going to teach me how to use the computer, or perhaps she would teach me how to work with one hand. Mark wheeled me in and parked me beside a table. There were no computers in sight. There were kitchen presses, and a large sink, and a kitchen chair. I saw a bath, and railings. It was an Alladin's cave of things. It must be a great fun- place to work in, I thought as I waited for the therapist to come along. Soon Ashling came in. She sat down and talked with me for a while, going through the period leading up to my stroke.

'Have you a good relationship with your G.P. Jean?' Ashling asked.

'I had a good relationship with my Doctor, Ashling, but I'm changing. I've been doing a lot of thinking about that subject since I've become ill, and now it's time for change.'

We talked about my home and who I had living at home with me. She set some tests to see if my sense of perception had been affected. I passed that test well.

'Is your husband supportive, Jean?'

'Yes, he's very supportive.' I answered. We continued to talk about how my illness had affected me, and how I was making progress so far. Ashling set more tests getting me to put a jigsaw together. I did it slowly, but successfully. She asked me to write my name. My writing was hardly legible. I told Ashling that I was feeling tired, and I needed a nap. She gave me another appointment for the next afternoon. Mark was called and he wheeled me back, going along the link again. Just then my friend Eithne arrived down to meet me. She had gone up to the ward, and was told that I was in physiotherapy, so she decided to come down rather than wait in the ward.

'Jean you're smiling,' she called out as we met. 'All that worried, frightened look is gone.' I introduced Eithne and Mark and all three of us went up to the ward.

When I looked around the ward I noticed a few new faces. Masie had been collected in my absence, and already a new lady was in her place sitting up, in readinness for her tests to start. At the end of the ward, near to the door a tiny woman had been put into bed. She could hardly be seen under the sheets. Nurse Rosemary was back on duty from her foreign holidays. She was golden, and beautiful and a little bit high. She was very taken with the little woman.

'You're a lovely little woman', she said to her as she passed by her bed.' I'm going to take you home, and put you on my mantlepiece.' The little woman buried her head further under the sheets. She smiled constantly, but she didn't speak at all. Again, when Rosemary passed by her bed she told her she was a lovely little woman. This time the little woman made a tiny sound.

'You'll be sorry.' She muttered.

Ciaran arrived in at seven. He brought cards from home, and flowers sent from my neighbours. Nicola arrived next, and before long Robert and Declan were there as well. It was good to see the children smiling at last. I knew it had been a very worrying time for them when I was very ill in the beginning. I asked Ciaran how Jessy was. She was fine. 'I'll head off early, Jean, Ulrica wants to get off early to-night. She needs a break from the house, and I have to walk poor old Jessy.' And off Ciaran went, kissing me good-bye before he left. He looked happier, too, to-day.

'Who is Ulrica, Mam?' Nicola asked.

'She's Dad's new housekeeper.' Declan informed her, both of the lads laughing.

'Has Dad got a housekeeper, seriously?' Robert asked.

'That doesn't sound right, Mam, Dad with a housekeeper, and especially one with a name like Ulrica. I think I'll drop in and see him to-night on my way home. I think Dad is really lonely, Mam. I wish you were home.' Nicola sounded worried. She kissed me goodbye and left to visit her Dad.

'Who is Ulrica anyway?' Robert wanted to know.

'She's Dad's new imaginery Swedish housekeeper.' Declan got great mileage out of Ulrica, but poor Nicola fell for it, hook, line and sinker.

Visiting time was over, and the drugs trolly came around. The nurses helped us into bed for the night. The television was left on for anyone who wanted to watch it for awhile. The ward was quiet without Masie. I spoke to the new patient in her place. She was in hospital for heart tests. She watched television before retiring for the night.

A new male patient next door could be heard giving trouble to the nurses. 'Give'is a cigarette, ah go on, just give'is a cigarette.' Staff nurse told him on no account would he get a cigarette as he was a very sick man, and that he couldn't smoke on the ward. He was going to be trouble. Sleep came easy after such a busy day.

Noreen could be heard laughing on her way next morning. 'Mornin girls,' she called out still laughing. 'The man next door asked me could he feel me wobbly bits,' she said giggling as she came in. She pulled out beds, and swept under them, and dusted and cleaned surfaces, happily going along, and never tiring. Her energy was amazing. When Noreen was emptying baskets of wilted flowers I asked her if

I could have the empty baskets for flower arranging, for when I got home. I collected lots of very pretty baskets, and looked forward to being able to make up baskets of flowers again. I kept them under my bed.

Jack was the the name of the old guy next door. As soon as he had his breakfast the longing for a cigarette started. 'Go on outta dat give'is a cigarette will yis.' He went on. 'Yis took me cigarettes, yis took me matches, yis took me money, yis took everything on me, so yis did.'

'We put your pension book, and your personal belongings in the locker for safe-keeping,' Sister told him. 'The doctor will be round in a moment, and will be coming to see you.' All was quiet for ten minutes. Soon he started taking little walks. When the coast was clear he came to our door.

'You're not allowed in the ladies' ward,' somebody called out to him, and he shuffled back to his bed, but not before reaching for a bar of chocolate from the locker of a sleeping patient. He looked weary and bored in his new surroundings. Before long he was out on the corridor asking people passing by for a cigarette and a light. He was successful until one of the nurses came looking for him.

'Back to your ward Jack.' He was back for a while again.

'Do any of yis smoke in here?' He asked looking in through our door. None of us smoked in our ward much to his disappointment, or so we told him. 'I didn't think yis did.' He said in a mocking way. He made his way back to his bed again.

'Are ye married?' he howled at Sister. 'I'd say ye couldn't get a man. Sure you wouldn't know how te, how te make a man a cuppa tea. Yappin, yappin, yappin, that's all yis do all day is yappin. Yis wouldn't know how to do a day's work. Yis never did a day's work in your lives. So yis didn't'.

When I came back from therapy the little woman was more alert. When Rosemary told her that she was a lovely little woman again a tiny voice came up. 'You'll be sorry,' she uttered more seriously. 'You'll be sorry.' Again Rosemary told her that she was a lovely little woman, as she helped her put on fresh pyjamas. Suddenly a tiny hand came up and lashed Rosemary across the cheek. Tears welled up in nurse

Rosemary's eyes. One of her colleagues took over and finished with the pyjama change, and advised her to leave the ward. When she returned she calmly continued her work on the ward, making no further comment on the little woman.

When the ward was quiet nurse's aid, Irene came up to my corner and we sat and looked through shiny magazines. When I got tired of sitting in the wheelchair Irene helped me into bed for awhile, and when I needed to visit the bathroom Irene helped me out, and waited outside until I called out, 'ready for collection.' I looked forward to the time when I would be able to transfer onto the toilet seat myself, and be able to get back safely into my chair as well. Still, I was making great progress, and I continued to work hard at therapy. Irene and I became great friends, and also Karen, who were both nurse's aids in our ward. These girls worked very hard helping us patients with showers, and whatever other needs we had.

Irene called my corner 'the office,' and whenever the ward got very quiet, as sometimes happened in the afternoons, Irene came up and sat quietly looking at shiny magazines spread out across my bed. Often I sat with a newspaper at one side of my bed while Irene sat at the far side enjoying the warm sunshine on her back. Flowers adorned my windowsill, and magazines accummulated alongside. My facecloth hung on the warm pipes with my towel. It felt like home, especially when the bed was so very comfortable as well.

CHAPTER SEVEN

O. T.

It was now two months since I had been hospitalised, and the subject of going home was coming up quite a lot in conversation with the Occupational Therapist. From now on she planned to come up to the ward every morning to show me how to wash and dress with one hand.

I thought it an impossibility at first, but it wasn't. Ashling had clever ways round everything. I sat in my chair and, first reached down to wash my legs. I dried them, and moved on to wash my arms and hands. When I had completed the task of washing, it was time for dressing. Very quickly I got the hang of balancing carefully, dressing the weak hand first, and then pulling my clothes over my head. My weak leg was still heavy, and it was a real challenge to pull trousers up and finally be able to stand and pull them up to my waist. It was great to be gaining so much independence.

I was told to take care of my left hand. Still, sometimes it fell down, and it hurt quite a bit at the shoulder when that happened. When I was ready Phil arrived up with the wheelchair to take me down to physiotherapy. We chatted as we went along down our usual route. These March mornings were chilly as we approached the lobby.

Ashling told me she would take me home by taxi to see my house one day soon, and to see how I would be able to cope when I would go home. I made a drawing of the sitting room, where I might be able to sleep, and showed it to Ashling.

The physiotherapist talked, together with me and Ashling about my progress. She set me more muscle strengthening exercises. Some involved tying weights to my legs for me to lift them. I was beginning to see progress at last. I was shown how to take the side off the wheelchair, and how to transfer to the bench bed without help. Exercises were set and I worked away while the therapist worked with other patients. I enjoyed being in the gymnasium working towards recovery.

A man shared a double bench bed with me and on one occasion he fell fast asleep. He snored out loud and rolled over to my side of the bench. 'Move over to your own side of the bed and stop snoring.' I called over to him. He looked really surprised when he woke up. We both laughed about it. The patients called the therapists physioterrorists because they made us work so hard.

Going back along the link with Mark I remarked to him how the seasons had changed since I came to hospital. It was January when I was admitted, and snow flurries accompanied grey skies. Now it was mid-March, and everywhere outside looked alive with growth, and the promise of better weather. Mark made me laugh as we went along. The porters were great therapists in their own special ways.

When we arrived back to the ward the Doctor from the Rehabilitation Centre was waiting for me. Mark lifted me back onto the bed in his usual way; like a sack of potatoes. The Doctor examined my weak limbs for sensation. There was still no sensation, but I had just a little movement in my leg. So far I had none in my hand or fingers. He said that he would come back to see me in a few more weeks. As yet I was not ready for the Rehabilitation Centre. I was glad because I liked the routine in the hospital, and I had got to know all the staff, and I enjoyed working with them.

I asked Sister if the hairdresser could call to cut my hair. It looked a mess. She made the appointment for the next afternoon.

Nicola called in to visit after lunch. 'Mam your hair is a mess.' She said to me. She was relieved to hear that I was having it cut. I got a break from therapy, and instead Nicola wheeled me down to the coffee shop, and we had coffee and a chat.'Oh yeah, I heard all about Ulrica from Dad, and me going up all worried to see him. The boys got a great laugh out of that.'

'You shouldn't believe all you hear Nicola.' I said to her.

When we got back to the ward Lizzy had been brought back to the bed beside the door. She was out of isolation after suffering from MRSA. She was still coughing. A nurse brought her a little container to spit in. 'If you get any phlem up spit it in there and we'll send it to the lab. Elizabeth.' The nurse told her.

'I think I'm going to be sick Mam - all this hospital jargon.' Nicola said. 'I mean Mam how could you eat a bite of food after listening to that?'

'That's nothing Nicola, you'd want to listen to things like bed pans, commodes, diarrhoea, constipation, and more besides, oh and blood tests, and B.M.s.' I added.

'What are B.M.s, Mam?' Nicola asked looking bemused.

'They are bowel movements, for those of us lucky enough to have them.' I continued.

'What way is that bowel of yours?' She asked cautiously, knowing the difficulties I was having. 'Have they put up that remedy yet?'

'Today is the day for the remedy after visiting time and I'm dreading it.' I whispered to Nicola. After visiting was over and the ward was quiet the remedy arrived. It eventually worked, but not without a great deal of discomfort.

'You're very good Jean.' The nurse praised me. 'Grown men cry like six-month old babies having that done.' Afterwards I felt really better and I had a long nap to recover.

When I woke up my brother John was sitting with me. 'You were snoring your head off Sister.' He said. He had a big bag of grapes and pears for me.

'You must have known I needed those.' I said. I doubt that he knew what I meant at all. Being ill in hospital makes you feel worlds away from those up and well in the world outside. I appreciated my family coming to spend time with me. It's an effort for people to travel to hospitals and to find parking spaces, and then to have to walk long corridors to visit, but it matters very much to help a patient recover.

CHAPTER EIGHT

Going Out

The Doctor came with her team on her rounds. 'Jean how would you like to go out on a visit home next Sunday?' Dr Lawler asked me.

'I'd like to go, I think, Doctor.' I said, trying to imagine it all at once. Sister came and had a long chat with me after the Doctor had finished her rounds. We talked about how I would be able to transfer from the wheelchair onto the car seat. It sounded really exciting. The thoughts of being in a car again, and being driven away from the hospital filled my mind.

'Sister, we have a wheelchair at home. It's brand new. It belonged to my mother-in-law. She died just two months before I got this. We were going to give it away.' I told her.

'Don't give it away, Jean. Maybe it will be suitable for you. Has it got large wheels on the back, or small wheels?

'I don't know, Sister. I never looked at it. It was just put upstairs out of the way, and we thought we might donate it to some place.' My mind was a whirlwind of thoughts.

'Ask your husband to bring it in Jean, and we'll have a look at it.' The thoughts of me in Granny's wheelchair really drove it home to me that I was disabled, and that I was going to be pushed by my husband in his Mother's wheelchair. It all seemed so ironic. We bought it especially for Granny, and yet she hardly used it.

Now, I began to think seriously of being at home. In the hospital I rang the bell at night for a bedpan, and a nurse came with one. How would I manage to visit the toilet at home?

In the morning breakfast was brought to the bed. A nurse helped me out of bed, and into the wheelchair. Thinking about all this made me feel a little despondent, although I was pleased with the progress I had made since the beginning. I was no longer crazy; refusing to wash, and not wanting to give blood for tests, and being afraid of everything. Still I had hoped for more progress. I felt moody, and tried to push the thoughts of being disabled from my mind.

When Nicola came in to visit I asked her to wheel me down the corridor so that I could practise standing. I could stand up holding onto something. When we came back to the ward Ciaran was there waiting for us to return. I told him how I could stand up at last. I demonstrated standing up holding onto his hand. Lizzy's family was visiting her, and they all applauded me.

I told Ciaran about the plan for coming out. He and Nicola were delighted to hear that. I asked Ciaran to bring me suitable clothes, and a hat as it was still very chilly. I needed shoes. I still wore circulation stockings. They were really cosy too.

The hairdresser arrived. She wheeled me out to the bathroom and began working on my hair. It was a relief to see all the long hair gone. She gave me a lovely short style just the way I wanted it. I felt re-invented. When she wheeled me back to the ward the nurses called me Posh Spice.

CHAPTER NINE

Coming Out

It was a bright Sunday morning, and an ideal day for my first visit out of hospital. The priest came to our ward at seven-thirty with Communion. Breakfast was served soon afterwards, and showers followed. Now I was able to dress myself, and put on my shoes. I put on my face, and I practised speech and facial exercises. The problem of dribbling had ceased, and my face looked normal again. The facial exercises worked very well.

After lunch Ciaran and Nicola arrived with the wheelchair from home. My jacket and hat were in it, and I was sitting waiting to go. The nurses helped me into the wheelchair, and wished me well going off. We set off on the usual route down the elevator, along the link, and instead of turning left for the gymnasium we turned right and headed out of the front door towards the parked car. The sun was shining brightly, and it was a crisp day. Nicola and Ciaran were smiling as Ciaran opened the car door. I was looking forward to showing off my skills at transferring from the wheelchair. I removed the side and easily slipped my bum onto the car seat. 'That's great Jean, that wasn't hard at all.' Ciaran said as he folded the heavy wheelchair and lifted it into the back of the car. 'That's a heavy bitch of a wheelchair; we'll have to get you a lighter one.' He commented.

'You're doing great, Mam.' Nicola praised me as we moved off away from the hospital.

'Would it be okay if we didn't go home to-day for my first visit, and instead maybe we could go to the Botanic Gardens?' I asked. I just wasn't ready for the emotional meeting with Jessy, my lovely Shetland Collie dog. Whenever I thought about her, and how she must be wondering why I vanished out of her life, it brought tears to my eyes. I needed to get a bit of emotional strength back before I was ready for home. I wasn't ready for any kind of emotional turmoil just yet.

'That's fine, Jean. Would you prefer to do that?' Ciaran said. 'And maybe next Sunday you'd like to come home for lunch?' It was settled. We drove along Dorset Street. I felt like an alien having just landed on earth. It felt more like years since I had been out in the world outside of the hospital walls. My head hurt at the slightest bump on the road.

'Are you alright Mam?' Nicola asked from time to time. 'You're doing great'. We reached Glasnevin in ten minutes or so. I felt quite fragile. Ciaran found a parking place. Again, he called the wheelchair a heavy bitch, as he took it out of the car. I got out with considerable ease, as I had been instructed by Ursula. We talked and laughed as we went along. Sometimes I thought how strange it was for Ciaran to be pushing me along. I thought of the many times we had walked here with the children; sometimes pushing one in a buggy, holding hands with each other; listening to the children searching for squirrels, and shrieking with excitement when they saw one. My emotions were raw. I felt happy despite everything. Nicola and Ciaran were full of cheer, and that was reassuring for me.

A man was being pushed in a wheelchair by a woman coming in our direction. I felt sorry for him. He didn't look old. 'Look at that poor man.' I commented thinking out loud. Suddenly I remembered that I, too, was being pushed along in a wheelchair. It was a raw reality. 'I'm being pushed in a wheelchair too.' I said surprising myself.

'Don't worry Jeannie. You're doing great. Do you remember how sick you were?'

'I don't want to remember.' I said. The gardens were bursting with Spring flowers, and buds looked ready to burst forth with blooms. It was fragrant, and fresh. Everybody looked peaceful walking along chatting as they viewed the lovely borders, and the variety of flowers. I spotted a man I recognised across the grass. 'There's Billy Heaney,' I remarked to Ciaran. He spotted us at the same time, and he and his wife made their way over to us.

'Good man Ciaran. I haven't seen you this long time.' Billy said in his usual friendly way.

'I haven't time to walk the dog these days Billy, between work and everything. I've been very busy.' Billy looked down at me, his hand reaching up to cover his mouth.

'What's this? What's this?' He commented taking a step back, and looking shocked, as he absorbed the change in me. I knew by the silence from Nicola and Ciaran that I would have to answer for myself.

"I had a stroke Billy.' I said. Then the tears started to flow. I felt horrified that maybe Billy might be upset. I knew he had had heart surgery, and I looked to his wife for forgiveness. 'I'm sorry.' I said floundering around for a way of escape. His wife came over and gave me a hug reassuring me that everything was alright.

'Poor old Jean had a very bad stroke about three months ago, and she's a bit shell-shocked. It's her first trip out of hospital to-day.' Ciaran said searching his pocket for a white handkerchief to mop up my tears. 'Do you know Doreen, Jean, Billy's wife?'

'How do you do Doreen?' I felt relieved now that that first meeting was over. I had not anticipated meeting some-one I knew on this trip out. Up to now I had not thought of my stroke as anything other than a severe illness which I was going to recover from. Now I was coming face to face with the reality of my situation. I couldn't walk, and maybe I would not be able to walk much again.

We continued walking for awhile. 'It was so difficult for me to say the word stroke. I have never referred to this condition as a stroke. I have no experience of saying stroke.' I confided to Nicola. The tears poured, and when they stopped they started again just as quickly.

'Could we go back to the hospital now, and maybe we could go to the coffee shop, and have a cup of coffee and relax there for awhile?' I asked. We continued back along the herbaceous border, each of us with our own thoughts and fears. Soon we were back and unloading again. The coffee shop was cosy, and before very long our spirits lifted. They both praised me at how well I coped with my first outing. That brought more tears. We went back up to the ward at five o'clock. Ciaran went home to feed the animals.

'Ulrica needs a break too, Jean. She's been stuck in the house all day you know.' He joked as he mopped my tears before leaving. My corner felt cosy with magazines on the window-sill, and my face cream and hand lotion on the locker beside my bed. Get Well cards covered a shelf above my bed, making my corner look colourful and furnished. I told Nicola that my bed was the most comfortable bed in Ireland. After Nicola left the tea was served.

Jack was quietly agitating for cigarettes. He followed Delia around the ward helping her gather up the trays after tea. His manner was improving towards the nurses. Delia allowed him help her collect dishes and it broke the monotony for him.

The trolley with the drugs came after our cup of tea at nine, and I fell asleep quickly, pulling the sheet over my eyes to hide the tears, which just kept pouring every time I thought about the day.

As soon as I woke next morning a lump came into my throat again. Ashling arrived to oversee my dressing. It was time to learn how to put on my brazier the easy way. I learned quickly, but as soon as Ashling asked how my outing went I broke down. 'Oh Ashling, I can't stop crying.' I confided to Ashling. 'It went well until I met someone I knew and then I got all upset.'

'It's alright to cry, Jean. If you didn't cry I would be more concerned for you. Is this the first time you've cried since you've had your stroke?'

'It's not my stroke, Ashling. I don't want it. I just don't want it any more. It's not fair. It's just not fair. I can't do anything. I can't even go to the toilet on my own.'

Ashling phoned the gymnasium and put my appointment forward till ten o'clock. She pulled in a chair, and talked and reassured me. She praised all my hard work so far, recounting how I was now able to sit upright in the wheelchair without falling to the weak side, and how I was able to go out of the hospital and have an outing. I felt better, and I washed and put on a little make-up.

Mark called to collect me. 'Are you alright young one?' He joked as he placed the pillow under my weak hand. Off we

37

went to the elevator. 'Were you out yesterday?' Mark asked casually while we waited for the lift to come up.

'I was.' I said cautiously. The lump started again in my throat. He pressed the bell, and we waited . 'We went for a walk to the Botanic Gardens.' I continued.

'Very nice. And did he bring you out for your lunch?' Mark teased.

'No. I had lunch here, and then we went out.' I said.

'You mean he didn't take you out for your dinner, and you had your dinner in this place. What! The mean so-and-so? That's terrible.' Mark had a wicked grin on his face, and I knew he was teasing me. Tears and laughter started all at the same time. Mark was cajolling me, and I had to laugh at his witty ways.

When we arrived in the gymnasium, Mark parked me beside the bench-bed. I took the side away from the wheelchair, and moved my bottom across, and onto the bench without any help. I felt pleased despite everything. As soon as Ursula asked me about my trip out the same outpouring of grief came, and she pulled the curtains around the cubicle while we talked.

Before long we got started and worked hard again. Today I was learning how to go up steps. The strong leg went up first followed by pulling up the weak leg. Coming down the weak leg was dropped first while the strong leg did most of the work, with the strong arm holding tightly on to the rail.

After lunch the nurses helped me back into bed. I was completely worn out from all the emotional turmoil. After a long sleep I woke feeling much stronger, and I was able to enjoy the company of my visitors in the evening.

Nurse's Aid, Karen was on duty, and when the ward was quiet after tea she came up to my corner for a visit. Karan was like a mother and a sister and a doctor all rolled into one. She was a great healer of the spirit. All the patients called on Karan for help, and she willingly helped with showers, or just about anything we wanted done. This evening she talked me through my emotional healing as well as my physical healing. 'It's all coming together, Jean,' Karen reassured me, and I knew she was right. Bit by bit healing was taking place. 'You are much stronger now than you were at the beginning, Jean. You can wash and dress without help from us. You are able to go out in a car. That's a lot of progress Jean.' Karen made us a cup of tea before going off duty for the night.

CHAPTER TEN

Moving on

I awoke fresh and energetic after so much rest. Irene helped me with my shower, and I set about getting dressed myself before Ashling arrived to help me with dressing. The morning sunshine filled my corner. It felt warm and I was happy again.

'How did you manage to dress yourself without any help?' Ashling inquired, as she entered through the curtains around my bed.

'I managed bra and all.' I boasted to Ashling. She had a look of surprise on her face. As I applied my face cream I heard the hospital shop being pushed through the ward.

'Could I have a mirror please?' I called out from behind the curtains. Ashling's mouth opened wide. She looked puzzled. I slipped a fifty pence piece under the curtain and a paper was passed under to my waiting hand. She thought I was calling for another mirror to look into. We both laughed about that.

Exercises got harder in physiotherapy, and I could see my progress now. The therapists were changed, and now I had a new physiotherapist looking after me. I liked Nuala. We were working to get me to lift my weak foot, and to move forward. My ankle was weak, and my foot flopped when I tried to lift it. Nuala presented me with my very own tripod. I felt really proud of it. Plans were made for me to go out again the following Sunday

Back in the ward Jack was giving trouble. When I returned he was missing from the hospital. Irene had been sent to try to find him. He was found standing out on the steps of the hospital begging for cigarettes. People gave the poor frail-looking old man a cigarette and lit it for him. Irene brought him back when he had finished smoking. He was only back a few hours when he went missing again. This time he couldn't be found, and the police were informed of his disappearance. He was returned late in the evening by the police, having been found in Temple Street in a house sipping tea.

He was no sooner back than he started giving trouble again. 'Go on outta dat give'is a cigarette. Yis wouldn't know how to make a man a cuppa tea. Yis never did a day's work in your lives. Yappin, yappin, yappin is all yis do is yappin all day. I'm gettin outta dis place so I am.' Sister was close by, and she was not pleased at his tone.

'What did you tell the guards when they asked you where did you want to be taken? Back here to the Mater isn't that right?' That kept him quiet for a while. As soon as Sister was out of sight Jack shuffled to the adjoining door of the ladies' ward. An elderly patient had several bars of chocolate on the top of her locker. His hand quickly picked them up and he slipped them into his pocket and he shuffled back to bed.

Some time later Irene wheeled me out to the bathroom to visit the toilet. There was a lot of noise and water splashing in the shower close by. It was one of the nurses showering Jack. 'I'm all wet. What are ye doing?' He bellowed.

'I'm washing the shit off the backs of your legs. Just shut up and don't be making noise. What were you eating that made you so sick?' I rang the bell when I was ready for Irene to collect me from the bathroom. There was so much noise coming from the shower room I doubt that they were aware that anyone had come and gone, and had heard them. The chocolate hadn't agreed with poor old Jack. Irene pushed me back to my corner.

Delia allowed Jack help her collect the dishes and trays after tea. It was to be his last day. He was being sent to a nursing home to be cared for next day. We became fond of the old fella despite his boldness. We imitated him at times, 'givis a cigarette outta dat. All yis do is yappin, yappin, yappin. Yis took me money. Yis took me cigarettes. Yis took everything on me so yis did.'

CHAPTER ELEVEN

More Outings

Talk was going round that nurses were being recruited from the Philipines, to fill the shortage of nurses at the hospitals in Ireland. There were more and more nurses returning to work in their mid-years, after rearing their children. When a nurse from the ward was absent through illness, or for some other reason it created a problem. Sometimes a nurse from our ward was asked to go down to help in Casualty, or to help in the renal ward. It was fine when the ward was quiet, but when our ward was busy we needed our nurses here.

We had a new nurse on duty. She was aged abouty sixty. She wore a nurse's uniform straight from the fifties. It had a wide flared skirt. Her name was Nancy. Nancy had spent several years working in South America, and she was a Nun. She just didn't fit in. We were glad Jack was gone. At least we didn't have to worry about him asking for a 'fuckin' cigarette,' and giving us all heart failure in case she heard a curse. I called her " Consuela." She had a most unusual accent. She spoke with a broken- English and Spanish accent.

The old lady in the bed beside me passed away in her sleep. As soon as the bed was changed and washed and dressed it was occupied by Betty. Betty was plump and she was a real giggler. When she laughed her whole body heaved, her face went red, and her shoulders shook. There wouldn't be a sound coming from her. I was glad to have Betty beside me. When I told her I called Nancy "Consuela" Betty shook with laughter. When "Consuela" entered the ward Betty's shoulders started shaking. She was a hopeless giggler. She just turned around in bed so Nancy wouldn't see her. When Nancy saw me apply fresh lipstick she said, 'you are beautiful.' This really made Betty shake. I knew she was giggling, even if she wasn't moving. After Nancy went back out to the nurses station, Betty mimicked what she had just said, copying her accent, and this got me laughing as well.

'You are beautiful.' And then she would shake all over.

We also had a nurse's aid on loan from another ward. She was enormous, and when she came over to help Betty she would sit on Betty's bed to have a little rest. The bed was hardly able to hold both of them. Betty told me she called her "Atilla De Hun." This set me off giggling again. Because Betty was a new patient "Atilla" offered to help her frequently. When I was having a cup of tea "Atilla" suddenly arrived in to offer help to Betty. When I saw Betty's face turning red I felt the giggles starting. I tried hard to stop, but the tea went up my nose, and made me cough and laugh out loud. The nurses hurried in quickly. 'Is there somebody crying in here?' they asked.

Our new batch of night nurses included Gillian with her black pony tail swinging from side to side as she walked through the ward. Her dimples and winning smile lifted our spirits. Denise, her friend and colleague was also back on duty after a week off. We felt in good hands when this strong pair of nurses were on night duty. Katie arrived in next, and they set to work preparing us for bed. I asked Katie how things were going with Gillian's Cork connection. She told me it was going strong, and she told me to ask Gillian about the milk quota. 'Yer man is always talking about the milk quota.' She told me. When my turn came to get into my pyjamas the craic started.

'Aren't you lucky to have such a lovely husband, Jeannie.' Gillian remarked, having just said good-night to Ciaran, as he left. 'Tell us Jeannie are you still in love as much as ever?' She asked as she shoved my weak leg into the pyjamas.

'Yes. I suppose I am.' I said. Her eyes looked dreamy as she pondered the thought. 'From what I hear you're doing alright yourself Gillian?'

'What do you mean, Jeannie?' She became suddenly alert.

'What about the farmer down in Cork then? Eh? Tell us about this fellow down in Cork Gillian.' I prodded her.

'Who told you that Jeannie? Did you hear us talking when we were going round the ward? Go on tell us or we'll tickle you, won't we Denise?' Denise smiled in agreement 'Come on mean Jean, on with your pyjamas.'

'And what's all this about the milk quota?.' She was going mad wondering how I knew.

'Who told you that? Was it Emma? If you don't tell us we're going to tickle your feet, aren't we Denise?' I wouldn't tell.

'You take that foot Denise, and I'll tickle this one. Are you going to tell mean Jean?' I laughed and laughed at the two big strong nurses tickling my toes when suddenly I felt sensation in my weak foot. I was so excited.

'Stop stop. I have sensation in my foot.' At last I could feel something after all this time. We talked for a while and then the busy nurses were on their way to settle the next patient down for the night. Next morning I was thrilled to be able to report the good news to my psysiotherapist, Nuala. I worked harder in therapy now that I felt sensation. I was learning to walk with my new tripod. One therapist helped to raise up my foot with a band tied around my toes, and the other girl helped me to move forward holding me round the waist.

'Tripod forward, right foot, left foot.' Nuala said, as she encouraged me forward, while the other therapist raised my weak foot with the band around it. They both worked hard and had incredible patience. 'Tripod forward, right foot, left foot,' and we moved another step. 'Tripod forward, right foot, left foot,' and we moved yet another step. The porter was asked to bring my wheelchair over to let me sit down. It was exhausting work. I wanted to do better all the time.

Mark wheeled me back to the ward. 'You're making great progress young-one.' Mark said as we went along the link. 'Soon you'll be going home.'

'I'm going home next Sunday for lunch, and I'm going to stay out a little longer this time.' I told Mark. When we arrived back in the ward I stopped to say 'hello' to Lizzy, and I introduced Mark while we chatted for a few moments. 'Lizzy has twelve children you know.' I said to Mark.

Mark started his dramatic usual self 'what! twelve children, what! My God you musta seen a lot of ceilings in your day.'

'Don't mind him Lizzy. He's very bold.' I said. Lizzy laughed heartily. Mark's cheeky ways often gave patients in the ward a lift. It was good to see Lizzy laugh again since her terrible sickness. Mark got to know the other patients when he was leaving me back every day.

I wanted help with washing my hair after lunch. Nancy offered straight away to help me. Betty was getting ready to giggle. I could see it in her eyes. 'Why are you in hospital anyway?' I asked Betty.

'I had a heart attack.' She told me. We had been so busy giggling that I forgot to ask her why she was ill. I got a right start to hear this. Now I really was wary that she'd laugh herself into another attack.

'You better stop laughing Betty.' I told her. Next thing Nancy arrived in with a hospital towel ready for hair washing. She wheeled me out to the bathroom, and gave my hair a good wash. 'Thank you Nancy.' I said, feeling a bit insincere. After towel-drying my hair she wheeled me back to the ward. I could sense Betty watching every move. I tried not to make eye- contact with her in case she would make me laugh again. Nancy went off to get the hair drier. As she blow-dried my hair she started at the base of my head and combed with her fingers going upwards as she went along. I glanced over at Betty. She was shaking; her shoulders heaving, and not a sound coming out of her.

'Now, you are beautiful,' said Nancy. I could see Betty lying down to hide the laughter. 'I'll show you yourself in the big mirror.' She wheeled me across the floor to look at myself. I could hardly keep my face straight. 'Now look, you are beautiful.' With that she wheeled me back to my bed, and off she went back to the nurses' station. Betty looked around at me.

'Am I like a hedgehog Betty?' I asked Betty, while I searched for my little mirror.

'No. You are beautiful.' And off we went laughing again.

As the week-end neared Dr. Lawlor asked me if I was happy about going out on Sunday. She said if it all went well they would allow me out for two days the following week-end. I discussed with her the trouble I was having with swollen fingers. I planned on having my wedding ring cut off, as it was impossible to move it. Perhaps I would ask my brother-in-law to do it for me. I trusted him as he was an engineer. That was agreed with Dr. Lawlor. And during this coming week I would be making a trip home with the Occupational Therapist to inspect my house. I was now into the fourth month in hospital. I got used to having my own wheelchair in the ward, and I started making short trips out the door, pushing myself along the corridor with one hand and one foot.

On one of my trips along the corridoor I was really surprised to see Kara coming towards me She was back in hospital, and coming to visit me. 'I can't believe that you're the same person Jean, you look so well.' I was so glad to hear that. Now I was up all the time, and out of bed. Kara told me all about her sheep dog, and about the farm and the Spring lambs. She was having her medication changed for her diabetes. And she was having some more tests done.

Our night staff were on in full force. 'Well are you going to tell Jeannie?' Gillian asked as she passed by my bed.

'What's a nice Wicklow girl like you doing going all the way down to Cork for a fella anyway?' I asked Gillian as she helped me on with my pyjamas. 'Tell me where are you from in Wicklow anyway Gillian?'

'Arklow, Jeannie. Why do you know anyone in Arklow?'

'Yes. I used to go out with a Guard, he is now stationed in Arklow. Patrick Killeen is his name. Do you know him?'

'You didn't go out with him? Did you hear that Denise? Jeannie had an affair with Paddy Killeen from Arklow.'

'Not an affair Denise, a romance.' I corrected.

'And where did you go dancing Jean? Denise asked, as we finalised preparations for bed.

'Well, Friday nights we danced in Mount Pleasant. We had a jar in the Charriott Inn, and on we went to check out the lads in Mount P.'

'I'd say you had a great old time. And where does your daughter go dancing?' Denise asked, as she helped me into bed.

'She goes to a place called Tramco. And where do you head off to when you go out galavanting?'

'McGowans in Phibsboro. Sometimes Roddy Bolands, and then again we head off into the city.' And off the busy nurses went to the next patient to prepare her for bed for the night.

CHAPTER TWELVE

Going home

Sunday morning I got ready to go home. I just couldn't wait to see Jessy. Would she run all around barking, or would she jump up on me in my wheelchair? When we arrived outside the house Ciaran unloaded the wheelchair and helped me out of the car. He opened the door, and Jessy came out yawning. She stretched first one back leg, then the other. I called her. She came over and sniffed at the wheels. Then she just toddled off across the road to the grass. 'Well that was a great welcome home Jessy,' I told her when we all got inside. It took about an hour before she became friendly with me.

It all seemed so strange to sit at our own table again. I began to feel sad at how I could not get up and walk as I felt I should be doing. The reality of being disabled hit home hard with me again. After dinner a terrible sorrow began to come over me, and great howls of crying poured out from the depths of my being. Tears flowed freely, and I didn't try to stop them, remembering what Ashling had said about crying. At about four o'clock in the afternoon I wanted to go back to the ward when I needed to visit the bathroom.

'Mam, I'll help you into the downstairs toilet.' Nicola offered. With the help of Nicola and my tripod I managed to make a visit. When I was ready I called out.

'Ready for collection.' Ciaran came to collect me. I sat in the sitting room for a little while, and again I felt I wanted to go back. I felt the hospital was home, and I just wanted to go back there. That started another outpouring of sorrow. 'Will I ever settle down again when I do come home for good?' I asked Ciaran. Sorrow produced tearfulness like I had never before experienced. It came from the depts of my being. My lost arm, my lost leg, my breast without sensation, my face frozen solid, made me cry, and cry until my eyes hurt from rubbing them.

'Of course you will Jean. Get them to show you how to peel potatoes in there, and you'll soon settle down when you start cooking the dinner again.' Ciaran joked. He went out and pottered in the front garden for a while. One of our neighbours, Mary, stopped to ask about me, and Ciaran invited her in for a chat. It was good to hear about what was happening in the neighbourhood. I told her how I was progressing along, since the day I was carried out of the house on a stretcher. She told me that everyone was shocked at what had happened.

After tea Ciaran agreed to take me back to the hospital. When I got back I wished that I had stayed at home, and the sad, unsettled feeling hung over me again. My head pained and a junior doctor was called to see me. 'You're getting the ugly one to-day,' he joked, explaining that he had been caught up in a rugby scrum. And he was ugly. His face was covered in bruises and scratches. He checked in my eyes with a light, and found nothing wrong. As long as the blood pressure was well down he was satisfied that all I needed was a good night's sleep.

Next morning I felt much stronger, and I knew that I was succeeding in making the break from the hospital. Dr. Lawlor came to visit me, and she told me that I could go out on Saturday next, as well as Sunday. Soon I was down in therapy working hard with Nuala. Together the physiotherapists got me into a standing position and one lifted the left foot while the other helped me to go forward with my tripod. 'Tripod forward, left foot, right foot.' Said Nuala, 'and again.' I was getting further away from the bench bed. Then we turned, and walked back again.

During the week Ashling came up to take me to visit my home as planned. She wheeled me down to the waiting taxi. Another staff member came along with us to help. Home felt a little more familiar now. Jessy was more friendly with me. Ciaran was waiting to let us in. Ashling planned where my bed would go in the sitting room when I was released home. We had a downstairs toilet, and that was a bonus. Initially I would need to have a commode, as I would have to transfer from my wheelchair. So far I still needed help going to visit the bathroom in the hospital. Also I had to be accompanied by a staff member in case of an accidental fall. The nurses explained to me that they would be held responsible if I had an accident. I was very careful I didn't want any more trouble to deal with.

Ciaran showed Ashling his fish pond in the back garden with the colourful Koi fish in it. On our way back to the hospital Ashling talked about the fish. The taxi driver told us he had a fish at home too. He said she was a pirranah. Ashling innocently asked him where he kept it. He told her he kept her tied to the kitchen sink.

Next day I had to make another trip out of the hospital to visit the dentist. Irene took me out by taxi. Going out and about began to feel a lot easier, and I looked forward to going out now, especially as the May sunshine felt warm and pleasant. I had been having pain in my left jaw. Although my face had no sensation in that side there was pain in the back teeth.

Sister checked in advance with the dentist if there was a downstairs surgery, as I would not be able to go upstairs. There was a downstairs surgery which was used for people with disabilities. My dentist found nothing but a tender gum, and he prescribed a cream. It soon settled down again.

Saturday came, and Irene helped me to shower and dress. I did my facial exercises in the ward. All was quiet at the weekends, and it gave patients a chance to relax and watch a bit of morning television. After lunch Ciaran called to bring me out to Stillorgan. Before we went there he first took me to see the Rehabilitation Centre. It felt very far away from home, and now I hoped that I wouldn't get a place there. We then went to have my wedding ring cut off. Brian, my brother-in-law, had the necessary tools for cutting. I was wary, but he worked away, and managed to cut my ring through. We had tea with Brian and Jo, and then we drove home to spend time with our own family.

We talked about how we would manage when I would be released home for good. The children assured me that everyone would help. We talked, too, about possibly building on an extra bedroom downstairs. The idea of going home now was sinking in with me, and I felt ready.

'Mam, I'll wheel you out in the park when I'm off work at the weekends.' Robert promised.

'And I'll take you round the supermarket if you want to buy any make-up or anything.' Declan added. So far I was sure of getting fresh air and hand lotion.

Sunday morning Ciaran called in really early for me. 'Mind the bumps,' I said as we went along. Every bump still hurt my head. We had invited Nicola and her friend Therese for Sunday dinner. Ciaran cooked a roast joint, and we ate and sat talking for ages. I stayed for tea and Ciaran took me for a walk around the Dublin City University close to our home. He sat on a bench, while I sat in my wheelchair, and we chatted in the glorious evening sunshine. A beautiful fragrance of fresh shrubbery hung in the air. I felt very happy and peaceful in myself.

Later in the evening he left me back to the hospital. This time I felt happy and I had no feelings of sadness. At last I was making emotional progress, and I was, at last, losing the need to go back to my bed in hospital. My thoughts now were of home and Jessy and family life.

The fact was that I had become institutionalized, and when I identified the problem I started learning to deal with it.

During the week I continued to work hard having weights tied to my weak leg to help strengthen the muscles. Dr. Lawlor came to see me before she went on holidays. 'Jean, you are our star patient for the year two thousand. You have made more progress than we ever expected you to, and you have done all the hard work yourself. Soon you'll be able to go home for good.' She said as she stood around with her team.

'Thank you Doctor Lawlor.' I said, 'but you have all worked hard to help me, and I appreciate it.' The following week-end I was scheduled to go out again, and I was looking forward to being out in the fresh air once more. May was a beautiful month with the shrubbery flowering outside in the hospital gardens. I continued seeing the therapists every day.

Karan came to sit with me for a while in the afternoon. 'How did you get on at home this time? she asked. 'Everything is coming together for you, Jean, and you'll manage when you get home too. Maybe I'll come up to visit you when you are at home.'

'Would you Karen? That would be really nice. Trouble is I might be tempted to ask you to help me with hair-washing, or nail-clipping, or God knows what.'

'That wouldn't be any trouble to me, Jean. I'm going to London to study nursing soon, so I'll be leaving here in a few months. I'm going to England to study for the next three years.'

'You'll be missed terribly here you know.' I said to Karen. I was quite surprised that she was leaving Ireland to study abroad, while there was a growing need for nurses in our own hospitals. 'Good luck to you, Karen, and mind yourself with all those lovely Doctors, and do come back to Ireland.'

CHAPTER THIRTEEN

Time to go home

Dear Diary,
I can go home next week. I will need a bed brought down to the sitting room. I'll also need a commode for use in the short term. Meanwhile I'm allowed out this coming weekend.

On Saturday morning Ciaran called to collect me at eleven o'clock. I was dressed and waiting to go home, and I was looking forward to getting away from the hospital environment, and to going out into the lovely fine weather again.

Once at home I picked up the phone and rang some of my friends and family. My friend Moyra offered to come to take me out for a walk in the park. I agreed, and she arrived up in the afternoon and off we went. It felt great to have someone to push me out. We went down through the park and on to her house not far from there. She helped me up the doorstep and inside. We had coffee and a chat. I felt perfectly normal. I didn't feel like a disabled person at all. Then Moyra helped me up and out to the wheelchair. She pushed me back up through the park. Along the route we met a mutual acquaintance. This person greeted Moyra, but she didn't look down at me. It amused me a little. 'Is this how we see people in wheelchairs?' I commented to Moyra. 'We don't see them at all; they're invisible!'

I felt like a wheelchair spy. From that on I observed people's reactions as we went along. I thought of my own reactions before I came out in a wheelchair. I couldn't remember; tiredness came over me as we neared home. I thanked Moyra for being my 'pusher.'

Right from the beginning I thought I would be able to walk again. I was pleased with my progress, but I wished I could put on my high heels and go places. I wanted to shake off the shackles of stroke, and get up and go. I had a beautiful dream that night of running around the park with the dog, and I wrote the following poem:

DREAM WALKING

I can walk in my dreams
Regardless of stroke
No wheels do I need
And my stick I can throw

I can go to the park
To the shops if I wish
And walking feels good
It's natural that's it

I can walk in my dreams
I can go skipping along
With the dog on a lead
And the cat running along

We go down the road
And we chat and we laugh
With the neighbours and friends
We know that we have

I can walk in my dreams
I've got get up and go
Just like I used to
Without props I can go

On Sunday Ciaran took me home again. It was a glorious day, and it made me want to be home permanently. I hugged him when we got inside the house. We were both very lonely, despite the fact that Ciaran visited me every evening, and twice a day in the beginning when I was acutely ill.

'I wish you were home for good.' He said as we sat down to Sunday dinner. 'Wednesday can't come quick enough as far as I'm concerned.'

'Ditto to that, same here.' I added

'I'm getting you a new single bed for the moment, and we'll put it in the sitting room by the window.'

'Oh good so. I'll be able to sit up and look out at the students going down the lane to the college. That's if I can stay awake long enough.' I said. 'And I'll be able to do some detective work as well. Any would-be burglars better watch out. And Jessy can sleep at the end of my bed.'

'We'll get there, Jeannie.' Ciaran added cheerfully. 'I'll be glad not to have to break my banjo down to see you every evening.'

After dinner we took a drive down to Skerries. Ciaran met someone he knew, and brought him over to the car to meet me. This time I was enthusiastic, and I swung my legs out of the car and stood holding on to the door, while Ciaran made the introductions. I shook hands with his old friend. My confidence was improving all the time.

Next morning Nuala made plans for me to be taken back for physiotherapy three mornings a week after my release from hospital. I would be collected by Johnny, the ambulance driver, at nine o'clock, and returned home afterwards. I was glad that I was going to have continuing contact with the hospital for awhile after going home. Now I was ready for this new challenge.

CHAPTER FOURTEEN

Home

Ciaran was an hour late coming to collect me. I was getting a bit agitated waiting and watching the door for him to appear. 'Sorry Jean I was waiting for the bed to be delivered.' He said as he hurried in through the door.

'This is one of the most important days of my life, and you are late.' I said. Not far away was Ashling and she heard me.

'That's not Jean I hear? Jean that's always so cool and calm.' Ashling remarked.

'I'm just a bit tense, Ashling. I better cool down.' And I did cool down. We went to the nurse's station to say good-bye to everyone. Irene was there. Her big brown eyes filled with tears that rolled down her face. I hugged Irene. She had always been so kind; helping me into bed, and then helping me up again, and always with a great sense of humour. Tears filled my eyes when I said 'good-bye' to the nurses whom I had got to know so well. Phil came in, and I said 'good-bye' to him too.

'You don't start crying, Jean or I'll start crying as well.' Phil said as he awkwardly backed away towards the nurses station. We left the hospital with my bags on my lap. My heart was heavy leaving all the people I had grown to love over the past four months.

Ciaran loaded my wheelchair and bags into the car. As we were driving away I discovered Betty. She was on her own smoking a cigarette outside the hospital entrance. She looked lonely and forlorn. She had been quiet all morning. I rolled down the car window and waved to her. 'You are beautiful.' She said, and her eyes filled with tears. I had to reach for a tissue when I remembered how Betty had been so much fun these last few days in hospital.

I promised myself I would settle down now at home, and I would continue with the exercise routine as arranged by Nuala. Jessy soon settled herself at the end of my new bed. I was able to wheel myself over to her and pat her while she dozed. 'Are you alright Jean?' Ciaran enquired from time to time.

'I'm fine. At last I feel at home. All the visits out of the hospital prepared me well for coming out.' I said to Ciaran. I pushed myself into the kitchen, and when I reached the sink I put on the brakes and stood up and pottered away washing a few dishes. 'What's for dinner?' I asked Ciaran. I pushed over to look into the fridge. He had the fridge full of fresh food. Ciaran cooked dinner that evening, but I was planning on taking up the cooking bit by bit, until I was able to cook as before.

I sipped a glass of wine. It was the first taste of alcohol I had in four months, and it tasted good. Ciaran slipped out to the local for a pint. I pushed myself over to see Jessy. She was already up on the end of my new bed curled up like a cat for the night. I buried my head in her golden fur. 'Did you miss Mammy when I was away Jessy?' She made a smug sound. She missed me. I prepared myself for bed feeling very pleased at how well the day had gone. Ciaran arrived back, and complained of being tired after a long and busy day. He excused himself and went up to bed. I felt a little sad that he didn't hug me, and tell me he was glad to have me home. I suppose he really was tired.

I pondered the thought of what change had taken place. I was no longer able to go up-stairs freely. Ciaran had been affected dreadfully, too, by my stroke. This past four months had been a terrible strain for him also. He had lost an able-bodied wife. He must have his own disappointing thoughts.

The sitting room looked really pleasant with the coal fire still burning red behind the fire screen. The heavy curtains kept the room warm and comfortable. I sat up in the darkened room and parted the curtains, and looked out at the world going by. A group of young people went down the driveway of the D.C.U. College singing 'The Fields of Athenry.' The Summer sky was a shade of dark blue. Suddenly flying across the tree-tops was Peter Pan and Wendy and with them was Ulrica. She was probably looking for a new job with some lonely husband. I slept well in my new bed.

In the morning Ciaran woke me with a cup of hot tea. 'Sorry about last night, Jeannie. I was just exhausted after running around all day.' He said. I put my arm around him and gave him a hug.

'Ciaran, I know this has all been a terrible strain for you too. My stroke has affected all of us, and not just me. I'm well aware of that.' I told him. And the children too, they must have been terribly shocked at the whole thing.'

'Don't worry Jeannie, we'll get there.' Ciaran reassured me. Some time later I wrote the following poem:

ALL YOU NEED IS LOVE

My love deserves a medal
For putting up with me
Every morning he comes down
He brings me in the tea

He never grumbles, never frowns
But always smiles while he's around
Though sometimes he gets cheesed off
When I'm behaving badly

There is a reason for this you see
It's the toe, the arm, the leg, the knee
I blame the weather, it's the cold
I say, and not me

All in all it's love I suppose
I cook his dinner, he washes my clothes
For better or for worse we wed
Thirty years ago that's what we said

I got worse
He's no better
But sure on we go
hell for leather.

On the first Monday morning Johnny called for me at nine o'clock. I was dressed and had my breakfast in plenty of time while I waited. Ciaran pushed me out to the waiting ambulance, and Johnny took over. He lowered a lever, and wheeled me on to it. He then raised it up, and wheeled me into the vehicle. After he secured the wheels to the floor he drove into the gymnasium.

The early morning was warm and the sun was bright and hazy. Johnny and I chatted as we went along. I enjoyed looking out at people's gardens, and I promised myself to get back to gardening as soon as possible. People were walking along wearing Summer clothes. It was good to be back out in the world again.

Nuala immediately got me working hard at muscle strengthening exercises. Ashling called in to see how I was managing at home. 'Everything's fine, Ashling.' I was glad to report. 'I'm even doing dishes standing at the sink, and I'm able to push myself over to the fridge, and take out food for cooking. Soon I'm going to be cooking the meals again.'

Nuala got me up walking with my tripod. 'Tummy tucked in. Bum tucked in. Head up, and look straight ahead.' And off we moved putting the tripod forward, then right foot, and then left foot, and we repeated the steps until we reached the far end of the gymnasium. Then we turned very slowly and returned to the bench bed. Nuala worked hard on my arm and hand. They were both becoming very stiff very quickly.

'Phil, where's Jean's chair?' Nuala was very busy to-day. Phil wheeled me out to the lobby to wait for Johnny. I pushed myself over to the florist's shop, and I sat looking at the fresh flowers and arrangements there while I waited. Outside, the sun was hot and the sky was blue. It was promising to be a good Summer. I was glad to be going out of the hospital, instead of going back up to the ward.

'We have two ladies to drop off first, and then we have one more call before we drop you off, Jean,' Johnny announced as we drove away from the hospital.

'Hail Mary, Holy Mary,' one old lady said when we reached the centre where they went daily. It gave me a shiver up my spine. Getting old is a scary thought. Johnny helped them down the steps, and they were met and brought indoors by a very kindly woman. Johnny told me as we went along that that old lady had a stroke, and the only words she ever spoke were 'Hail Mary, Holy Mary.'

And so for the next three months I went to the hospital gymnasium three mornings a week. I became much stronger. I was now able to get around the house walking a little with my tripod. I could get into the down-stairs toilet without any difficulty. Ciaran took me to visit family, and friends. I was enjoying life once again.

Karen, the nurse's aid from the hospital, phoned me to say she was going to come up to visit, as promised, on Saturday afternoon. I gave her directions. She said she would probably borrow her Mum's car. I was keeping an eye out for a small car stopping outside our house. I was most surprised to see a tiny girl arriving on a great big black motor bike. She was dressed in black leather wear, and when she dismounted she removed a great black helmet, revealing the lovely sweet girl that I knew from the hospital ward. She looked so different I couldn't believe my eyes. We had a cup of tea, and a great chat. She was surprised at the improvement in me in such a short time. Karen was leaving soon to study nursing abroad, and I wished her well. I have not seen her since.

Nuala sent me to have a special splint made to keep my foot from flopping. First a cast was made, and from that the specially-fitted splint was made to fit my foot. I was called for a fitting. It felt very comfortable, and my shoe was put on over it. I then had to walk between two bars holding on with my strong hand. The difference was amazing; I could walk much better wearing the new splint. When I went back to the hospital Nuala was very pleased. She then presented me with my very own walking stick. Nuala was leaving to go to Australia, and now I was passed on to a new therapist. On one of my next visits I was released fully from hospital with a programme of exercises to continue to do at home daily.

The letter came from the Dublin Corporation giving approval for a grant towards the cost of building an extention bedroom onto our house for me. Now, we could advise the builder to go ahead with the work. I was not looking forward to having the disruption of building work being carried out on my home, but we went ahead with the plans. The builders arrived with heavy equipment. First thing they had to do was to knock down the garden shed, and that meant a lot of noise. I asked my friend Grainne if I could come round to her house for a couple of hours during that first day. Ciaran dropped me off, and collected me in the evening on his way home from work. After that I phoned my sister, Helen and asked her if I could come to stay with them for a couple of days. Off I went with my bags packed for a nice little break.

My brother-in-law, Michael took us out for breakfast to the Square shopping centre in Tallaght. I had not been to this centre before, and it was a real novelty. As he unloaded my wheelchair I spotted a young woman driving a motorised wheelchair across the parking area. She was speeding along, and she looked really happy. She made a lovely picture for a person in a wheelchair. 'That's for me.' I said. I didn't think of her in a pitying way. 'I'd love one of those.' I said. 'I'm getting one of them.' From that moment I was really excited at the prospect of being able to drive myself to the local supermarket, and being able to do my shopping independently. I could go to Mass, and to the chemist. There were so many places to go. For now I was really enjoying being on a short holiday away from home.

When I returned home the foundations were in, and the men were working away. I was able to make tea and coffee for them whenever they needed it. The plans included a sliding door which I could use to drive out onto a slope. It was designed especially for my needs. I would also be able to do gardening, as the garden was a patio garden, with raised flower-beds. When the work was near to completion I would be ready to go shopping for a motor.

We had brick-layers, electricians, etc. etc. all working on my new room. It was fascinating to see the whole thing coming together. When the work was finished, and the builders left with all their equipment, I gave a sigh of relief that at last it was all done. Now it was up to Ciaran to put his decorating skills to the test and finish the look of this new creation. I was delighted at how it all turned out.

CHAPTER FIFTEEN

The Stroke Club

My new General Practitioner suggested that I join the Volunteer Stroke Scheme. At about the same time my daughter made contact with the Stroke Club, and asked if someone would call to see her Mum. The Supervisor made contact with me and we arranged a time for her to visit. I was able to open the door to Erica the Supervisor. We had a good chat. She had a great understanding of stroke and it's after effects. She made plans for me to be collected by a volunteer driver the following Monday. I went along and had a really good time getting to know other people with similar disabilities as mine. When I came home I wrote a poem about the experience.

FIRST DAY NERVES

My first day at the Stroke Club
It was an inspiration
I thought they'd all be old folk
From a different generation

Oh no indeed they weren't
A fit lot I could see
Telling jokes and stories
And as jolly as can be

There wasn't a complaint from one
Not even a little moan
The only sign of trouble was
When it was time for home

Then we all got up to leave
And out we wobbled slowly
Some with sticks or tripods
Striding forward boldly

We covered Summer holidays
Showed photos from a trip
Introduced ourselves around
A day without a slip.

And so, from that Monday on I have been going to the Stroke Club. I have made new friends with people with similar difficulties as my own. We plan our outings in the Club. Our first outing was to Dollymount House for Halloween. We had lunch followed by a fancy dress competition. Our volunteers dressed up, and helped us stroke people to dress in fancy dress, if we wished, and take part. Our inhibitions about our wobbly legs and our stiff arms and hands were soon forgotten, and we took part enthusiastically. The winner was announced, and a prize was given.

Our next celebration was the Christmas party. We were able to bring along a friend or family member. My daughter Nicola came along with me. Christmas dinner was served in the Club. We had a glass of wine to accompany it. Our volunteers put on a show after dinner with some of the stroke people taking part. It was first class entertainment. A musician was hired to play all evening, and before long we were up dancing; even those of us with weak legs. Yes, we were able to do the twist, and waltz with someone holding on to us carefully. Afterwards we had a bumper raffle. We sang Christmas songs. And when we were tired we were taken home by our volunteer drivers, or family members.

Every second Monday a physiotherapist comes to the Club to put us through a suitable exercise routine. It helps to motivate us to continue practising exercises at home. It's essential to exercise every day to keep stiffness at bay. It also helps prevent pain. What I discovered as time went on was an increase in pain along the stroke side. In the beginning there was no pain in the limbs, but it crept in by degrees.

For those of us who wear splints we can have difficulty with soreness in the toes sometimes. This comes from a build up of pressure. The splints are, after all made from a type of hard plastic. At the Stroke Club we are able to discuss these issues with other club members. I took part with others in research into different kinds of splints. That research was done in the Dublin City University.

Chapter Sixteen

My Motor

It saddened me greatly to see my lovely pet Jessy become unwell. She was aged thirteen, and had had a very good life; walking in the park every day, and being generally spoiled. Ciaran took her to the vetenarian. She was kept in overnight, and was put on antibiotics. A drip was put into her little leg, but they advised me that she was failing. Next day we decided to have her put to sleep.

It was time for me to move on. The time was right now for me to go shopping for a wheelchair. I phoned and made an appointment for the very next day.

I got an appointment for two o'clock. I was so excited I could hardly finish eating my lunch. Now I was really going places. I had an appointment with Alan, the salesman.

When I saw the array of scooters all lined up, gleaming, and all brand new I just couldn't believe my eyes. It looked like Santa's workshop. I wanted to try out all of them. Along came Alan. 'Well, what can I do for ye?'

'I want to look at motorised scooters and motorised wheelchairs.' I said merrily. He discussed with us the type of chair most suitable for my needs. I looked around and enquired about different models of chairs I saw. Some looked very big and elaborate. I wanted a trim-looking machine.

'What colour would you like, Jean?' Alan asked.

'I have no idea.' I said. 'It's not like buying a dress or a coat or something to wear. What colours have you got?' I asked him?'

'Well, we've bottle green or black, or would you like purple?'

'I think bottle green is a good colour on me. It's one of my favourite colours. Can I try one in bottle green so?'

Off Alan went and in a minute he arrived back driving a bottle green motorised wheelchair. It was a beauty. 'Now try this one, Jean.' He said. I gave my tripod to Ciaran to look after, and I got carefully into the beautiful wheelchair. 'Now, you follow me; out through dat door, alright Jean? Just press the joystick forward to go straight. When you want to go left press it towards the left, and right when you want to go right, and dat's all there is to it.'

I pressed the joystick, and straight away it moved forward. I was smiling all the time with excitement. 'O.K. are you behind me, Jean? You follow me, right Jean, down dat slope. Right de ya see dat wall down there, Jean? Right just go straight towards dat wall.' We were now outside. 'Dats it, good, go on, dats it, Jean. When you want to stop, bring the joystick back to it's normal position.'

'It feels great, Alan. I'm moving forward.' I was so excited I started laughing, and the tears streamed out of my eyes. I had to stop driving and get a tissue out of my pocket to wipe them. Ciaran was close-by. Alan looked back to see if I was following him.

'What's wrong? Is she alright?' He called over to Ciaran.

'She's just excited?' Ciaran said back to Alan, with a look of 'you know women', on his face. I moved off again, and soon began to feel more natural driving. And then I started to think of me going to visit Grainne. I could imagine Grainne opening the door, and being so surprised that she comes out with something outrageously funny. Away I started laughing again. I put my hand to my mouth to stifle the giggles. Tears poured down my face. My make-up was ruined. The wheelchair came to a standstill while I dried my eyes. The left hand cannot do anything, so stopping to use my right hand meant coming to a complete standstill. Soon I was away again in command.

'Now, Jean head straight back up towards the door. Dats it, follow me now and take a wide turn, and up the slope and carefully go in through the door.' And we got back inside. It was easy. 'Well do you think you could manage one of these things?' Alan asked me.

'Yes, I could. I'd be well able to manage this, Alan.'

We completed the paperwork, and the new wheelchair was to be delivered at three o'clock the next day. I went home brimming over with excitement. I could hardly wait till the following day for it to be delivered.

After lunch the next day I was watching the front room window. It was twenty minutes past the appointed time before the van pulled up. The two men got out and unloaded my wheelchair. They brought it to my back room and up the slope. My room was free of furniture while Ciaran was decorating it, and it was ideal for me to practise driving in before I ventured out. The joystick was sensitive to touch. I mastered the ability to drive it very quickly. I went out round the park with Ciaran. We had no dog now, but it felt good to be able to go out for a walk together, especially without Ciaran having to push me along.

My next trip was to the supermarket. I had no trouble crossing the dual carriageway. I just pressed the button, and waited for the green man, making sure that the traffic had come to a stop before I pointed my joystick forward, and off I went, being careful not to drive it into someone's heel. I could go into the chemist, and leave in my prescriptions for my medication. Before very long I was able to go to visit my General Practitioner for whatever needs I might have. A poem soon came to mind:

FREEDOM

I want to tell a story
About something I hold dear
It gets me out and about
It's my motorised wheelchair

I drive around the park
And chat to everyone
I go over to the florist
I can go anywhere I want

And I go to visit Grainne
And to Church to Sunday Mass
Grainne calls me Mary Poppins
Sure we always have a laugh

And I go down to the doctor
To get my prescriptions filled

I charge down through the park
Oh I love going down the hills

And I love the feel of freedom
That my wheelchair gives to me
As long it's not pouring rain
I'm as happy as can be.

I get great enjoyment from children's remarks when they see me in my wheelchair. On one occasion a small boy watched as his Dad helped guide me out past a big lorry parked, and blocking my way. The Dad beckoned to me to come on. The boy was thrilled looking at his Dad being such a hero. 'It's well for you. You don't have to walk anywhere.' He said delightedly. I laughed, but his Dad wasn't sure how I would take it. And on another occasion when I was going past the school a boy called to his friends. 'Move over and let the girl pass in her wheelchair.'

Grainne got a big surprise when I rang her door-bell, using my walking stick to press the bell. 'Here's Mary Poppins.' She said laughing, when she opened the door to me. It gives me great freedom to be able to go to all of these places, since getting my wheelchair.

We missed not having a dog on our walks in the park. I suggested to Ciaran and my son Declan that, perhaps, they would go to the dog pound and just have a look to see if they have any nice little female dogs there. I gave clear instructions that, on no account did we want a male dog 'going around thinking he owns the place.' Also, 'we don't want a black dog.' I didn't think I'd like a black dog for some reason. They went to the dog pound alright.

'Mam wait till you see this little dog. We can collect him tomorrow.'

'What do you mean collect him, Declan? I thought I said no male dogs.'

'Ah Mam, wait till you see him. He keeps wagging his tail. He's really a happy little dog.' I looked to Ciaran for an explanation. He just smiled looking helpless about the whole thing. And so, the next day they went to collect the little creature. I was having a lie on in bed, when they arrived in with the little black puppy. He jumped straight up on my bed, and lay down for a minute and looked quite at home. He is two years old now, and I wouldn't part with him for a million euros. We had no name in mind for a male dog, so we started at the beginning of the alphabet until we came to f.

'Flash, how about calling him Flash.' I suggested. And so it was, we called him Flash. He is a collie cross type dog and a great friend and protector.

As Ciaran was between jobs at the time he was able to take Flash to the park early every morning. Both of them came back breathless from the early morning air. Many other dog owners also walked their dogs, and Flash made lots of friends. Ciaran talked excitedly about Heidi every day when he came back from the park. Since I walked Jessy for all of thirteen years I knew that people formed friendships from meeting frequently in the park, and chatting casually. Eventually this prompted me to write a poem:

HEIDI

I have to meet Heidi
The mystery lady
With her black and white coat
I hear of her daily

How she runs with great speed
And she glides with great style
I've been hearing about Heidi
Now for quite awhile

She's made friends with himself
He's her great admirer
And she responds with affection
The beautiful Heidi

Flash likes her too
The two men in my life
But Heidi is lovely
And she causes no strife

She's owned by the Reverened
And his family and wife
The beautiful collie
That's Heidi.

It was time to type some of my scribbles into the
computer. Declan told me how I could down-load my 'stuff'
onto a floppy disc, and print it on his printer. And so I began
using the computer. Every few minutes I called him to find
out something I didn't know. He was going crazy telling me
how to do things, and five minutes later it had slipped my
mind. While I waited for him to return home to help me with
something I sat with pen and paper, and behold a poem came
to mind. I submitted it for the Valentine's Day poetry
competition at the Stroke Club.

I HEART THE COMPUTER - NOT

Learning the computer
It just would break your heart
Every time I learn a bit
I forget it just as fast

'I lost the text again,' I call
'Declan help me to recall'
'I've told you fifty times before
I'm not going to tell you anymore.'

'Enter here, save it there
No don't press that, here press this'
With computers there's just no bliss
Pen and paper for me that's it

'You have to learn, it's easy Mam
I'll help you out if I can
You must listen then you'll know
With your mouse where to go'

'Start again don't loose heart
Switch it on, there you are
Oh that's better there you go
The computer now you nearly know'

'How can I save it again?' I ask
Declan's losing patience fast
'I told you fifty times or more
I'm not telling you any more'
Declan calls going out the door

    I enjoy using the computer. The more I use it the more I become familiar with its peculiar ways, and the more I appreciate what marvellous things it can do. Declan has been great, guiding me along when I'm stuck, or when the computer acts up. I often wondered if he was badly shaken that morning I called him up five years ago. 'Declan did you get a terrible shock when I called you up the stairs that day when I had the stroke?' I ventured one day.
    'No, not really Mam. I didn't know what a stroke was. I never knew anybody with a stroke. I thought it was some woman thing or something. No don't worry Mam, it's cool.' He assured me.

CHAPTER SEVENTEEN

Life Goes On

For survivors of stroke life goes on. For some patients disability is very severe. Aids such as tripods and walking sticks are necessary. For patients who like to get out and about the motorised wheelchair is a great boost to confidence and the sense of independence.

When an illness occurs after stroke, such as an infection, the weak limbs become much weaker. A patient who is able to get about walking with the help of a tripod or stick now finds that the level of strength is greatly reduced. Walking can feel near to impossible. When the illness passes the strength returns gradually. These minor illnesses cause setbacks, and can be a huge disappointment to a patient, especially in the early stages of recovery.

Patients recovering from stroke need an enormous amount of support to boost the shattered confidence. A patient needs to be highly motivated towards recovery, and needs to have a strong desire to go on with life, despite the disabilities. This helps prevent depression from setting in and taking hold. A support group such as the Volunteer Stroke Scheme means a great deal to people recovering from stroke. Patients can meet in a club setting, and can enjoy activities together. Knowing other people with similar difficulties as yourself lessens the feeling of isolation. I am very fortunate to be living near to the Volunteer Stroke Scheme. Every Monday morning I am collected by a volunteer driver, and taken to the club.

We have a physiotherapist who comes into the club on alternate weeks. She puts us through a programme of suitable exercises. We are encouraged to do these same exercises at home to prevent stiffness and to help overcome pain. They work very well, and give one a feeling of well-being. We play bingo, skittles, darts, do flower arranging, hold quiz sessions, paint Christmas cards, and we do creative writing, also in the club. Tea and coffee starts the morning off, and chatter soon fills the place, and we end off the morning with a raffle.

Last year the club took thirty stroke people on a four-day holiday to Co. Clare. I was one of the lucky people to go.We were taken from our club, at St Luke's hall, by coach. The driver took us first to collect our south side friends from Mount Argus, where they were all waiting. Some had wheelchairs, and some more were standing outside with walking-sticks looking delighted to see us arriving to go on holidays. On the way we stopped for lunch. It takes all of us quite some time to visit the toilets after lunch. With the use of one hand only, opening zips and buttons takes time. As we strolled out to board the bus I noticed that the woman who was beside me on the coach was smoking a cigarette. I commented to her 'Ellen aren't you very bold to be smoking dirty old cigarettes after having a stroke.'

'It's alright, my doctor knows I smoke.' She replied, puffing away before she got onto the bus. We were just getting the last few people on board when suddenly Ellen stopped talking. I glanced sideways, and to my surprise Ellen had passed out beside me. I had to think fast. It was possible that she had had another stroke. I opened her blouse to let her breathe easily. I called the supervisor and a volunteer. Next thing her false teeth came out of her mouth. I reached across and picked them in my hand before they fell. Tess, one of the volunteers, had a tissue and she wrapped the teeth in it. Ellen would need them when she was well again. There was no improvement in Ellen, so we called an ambulance for her. It arrived quickly and the crew took her out and brought her off to Naas hospital. When they gave her oxygen, she began speaking in the ambulance. We set off minus our supervisor and one volunteer, Jim, who went in the ambulance with Ellen. We continued on our journey, and the sun shone brightly as we went along.

We stayed at the Auburn Lodge Hotel in Ennis. A number of volunteers came along to help, as well as our supervisors. It was a real treat to come down to the dining-room for breakfast, with everything cooked and ready to serve. After a little time to relax after breakfast, our coach driver helped us back onto the bus and took us out for an outing. We went to see Bunratty Castle, and the Folk Park. I particularly liked the Folk Park. We visited a house there where a woman showed us how bread was made in the traditional way, and how it was baked in a pot oven over a turf fire. We visited the farm with sheep and pigs and hens and a cockeral all lazing in the sun. News came that Ellen was recovering, and that she would be home in a couple of days. We were relieved to hear that she was going to be alright.

Our volunteers pushed those of us who were unable to walk very well in our wheelchairs.When the rain paid us a visit we made our way up to Dirty Nellie's Pub. A German tourist helped me down the steps. We relaxed there with a few jokes and a song, a glass of wine, and a few beers. Someone helped me back up the steps when it was time to join the rest of the group. It was a funny sight to see two wheelchairs parked outside of Dirty Nellie's Pub.

Next day we were taken to Lahinch, a beautiful coastal town. Our group had lunch in Lahinch, and we separated to go off shopping. Kitty and Tess, two of our volunteers, took turns in pushing me. We did a bit of shopping before joining the rest. With my two pushers we had plenty of laughs as we went walkabouts. We came back and watched the big waves breaking along the coastline.

When we returned to the hotel we had a rest period before dinner. The hotel provided us with a tray set with teacups and a kettle and milk, so that we could help ourselves to a cup of tea in our rooms on our return. My room mate Joan Kiely, made us a cup of tea when we got down to our room. Joan has better use of her weak hand than me. I slipped off my splint and shoes, and lay back in the bed for a rest before dinner time. We arrived down to the dining room for dinner at seven o'clock, and once again it was delightful to have beautiful food served up. This again gave all of us a chance to get to know each other, and with a glass of wine with dinner, we were all very relaxed. We sat back and swapped stories about the falls we had, and the times spent in rehabilitation etc.

Each evening there was entertainment after nine in the hotel, and we got right into the spirit of things. Our coach driver told us that he was a bit worried taking off with us, but he was really surprised at how well we were able to manage to get around. With our wonderful volunteers we had a lovely holiday in Co. Clare. We headed back to Dublin feeling relaxed and refreshed. We first dropped off the people from the southside of Dublin at Mount Argus. We had enjoyed getting together with the other club, and getting to know them.

There were very few complaints on holiday from my fellow stroke people. We have a good deal of pain to deal with in our affected limbs, but with daily exercise and a little pain relief we can deal well with it.

Once back from holidays I was full of enthusiasm for cooking and gardening and going places. Much is said about disability, but we hear less about ability. Indeed it is very important to focus on ability. In my case I shop for groceries, I cook dinner every evening. I can make most meals like curries, stews, omelettes and roast dinners. It took a while to get the hang of peeling potatoes with one hand, but once I got some practice I was soon able to peel them as quickly as one would with two hands.

We need to have a great deal of patience after stroke. Our families also need patience with us while we cope with the adjustments. For example, when I decide to go out somewhere I have to get my coat and put it on; starting to pull it on to my paralyzed arm first. It can fall to the ground if I'm not careful. When I'm ready to go out I get into my wheelchair, open the sliding- door, and I drive out into the garden. I lock the door, pulling it shut with one hand. I drive down the slope, and out through the side entrance. Again I lock the side door using one hand to do everything. The staff in my local supermarket, Eurospar, are very helpful, and I have no trouble shopping. I feel a great sense of achievement at being able to shop, and cooking gives me a good sense of being a useful person.

Another great achievement is being able to travel into the city centre on the bus. Thanks to Dublin Bus for making a special platform available on the buses for people using wheelchairs. We are able to drive onto the bus, and then park safely once inside. The bus then glides along, and it's easy to drive off again and go about your business in town like everybody else. Last Summer Ciaran accompanied me on my first trip to town. We got off the Nineteen A bus at Trinity College, and on a beautiful Summer's day we went up Grafton Street. I was fascinated at the street entertainers. The first one I saw, I stopped my wheelchair to look at him. He was standing looking like a statue, with not a move out of him. I watched, and watched, but no, he looked like a grey statue I began to ponder the thought that he might, indeed, be a statue. Ciaran moved on calling me to come along. I smiled at the statue-like man before I left, and waved him goodbye. His hand moved and he waved goodbye to me. I just laughed and laughed. There were several more entertainers along the street. We continued on along until we came to St Stephen's Green. We went around the park and enjoyed looking at the flowers there.

Every month I go to a book club in my local library. The library is wheelchair-friendly, and I have no trouble going in or out of it. I also attend the U3A group in the Ballymun Library. This group is for older people. It is called University for the Third Age. It is not a University, but a gathering of older people who meet and take part in activities together. It is learning in an informal way. We have people who come to give talks on various subjects. For example we had a man who gave a talk on the History of Glasnevin. It is a relatively new group, and I'm just beginning to get into the swing of things there. We have a trip to Cork planned, and I'm just trying to work out how I might be able to manage if I go.

All the paths in my area are wheelchair- friendly; a must if you need to drive down off the paths and continue on your way. I can go to the chemist locally for my needs. The paths are wheelchair-friendly all the way to the Botanic Gardens, another place Ciaran and I like to go to visit occasionally There is a slope going up to my Church for use for buggies or wheelchairs. If I need tickets for the Helix, that too is also suitable for me, and I can attend a show there, sitting in my wheelchair. That brings a poem to mind:

EURO STAR

Oh, it was a noisy night
That's what I remember most
But a special night it was
The semi-final of the Eurovision song contest

'Mickey Joe' they shouted
From everywhere around
And the youngsters whistled loudly
Sure you couldn't hear a sound

And when Mickey Joe came on
You could hardly hear his song
And they quietened down a bit
When Mickey Joe was done

When the lads were finished singing
One of them had to go
Leaving two to compete
At the next Sunday's final show

Oh. The songs were very lovely
Michael, Simon and Mickey Joe
They did a splendid job
It was a very enjoyable show.

It is very important for stroke patients to be encouraged towards independence. Simple everyday- tasks such as tying your own shoelaces with one hand is easy when you know how. If this was done for a patient out of kindness then that person might become dependent on having it done for them every day. This is usually taught to the patient while in hospital recovering from stroke.

The occupational therapist in your area can be contacted long after release from hospital to help with working out problems as they arise. For example a second stair rail is necessary for going up and coming down stairs safely. In recent times I had one such job done by the Health Board in my area. It is vitally important for us stroke people to avoid falling. I've had a few falls, and fortunately I escaped injury. It brings to mind the last Valentine's Day outing we had with the Stroke Club to Forest Little Golf Club, and the usual poetry competition:

This was my entry:

MY VALENTINE

My Valentine is ever patient
And he is always there for me
It's been five years since my stroke
And he's still as good as he can be

He's a kind of fortune teller
He knows things in advance
'You'll fall if you're not careful'
He said, giving me a sideward glance

He took the dog out for a walk
Before he went to bed
I went to spend a penny
But I fell across the floor instead

My hand it hit the ground
At an awful speed
I just sat up and checked around
There was no pain, there was no bleed

'You're lucky you didn't split your head
Or crack a hip,' that's what he said
'You could have been another statistic
Waiting for a hospital bed.'

'I fell for you again that's all
It's Valentines night if you recall'
He helped me up and into bed
Good night folks, there's no more to be said.

CHAPTER EIGHTEEN

Stroke Prevention

Some time ago I was asked by a pharmaceutical company to speak to a large group of doctors about my personal experience of stroke. It was in connection with the launch of a new drug for treating high blood pressure. In advance of this I made some notes to remind me of what I wanted to say. One note was: 'Doctors don't let your patients have stroke.'

General Practitioners are first in the line of fire when dealing with our health problems. This puts them in a very responsible position. We depend on them to deal with serious problems, such as high blood pressure. There are other serious illnesses such as diabetes, high cholesterol, overweight, and previous mini stroke, or transient ischaemic attack, to be taken into account to prevent serious strokes. And there are hereditary factors to be taken very seriously in stroke prevention.

As time has gone by since my stroke I have read quite a few articles and books about stroke. There is not very much written by Irish people who have been severely disabled by stroke. I picked up a little information along the way.

Much needs to be done to prevent strokes. Statistics show that nine thousand people suffer a stroke in Ireland every year. One third of these strokes cause death. The rest cause a wide range of disabilities. This puts a huge financial strain on the Health Board. There is enormous loss in terms of productivity and contribution to the economy. But the greatest loss of all is the loss to the patient who suffers a stroke, and to his family.

The incidence of TIA, or transient ischaemic attack needs particular attention. When a TIA or mild stroke happens a person is at great risk of suffering a further stroke at a later stage, unless the cause is investigated and treated, and the patient's health is monitored carefully by a General Practitioner.

According to statistics there are thirty thousand people in Ireland, at the moment, disabled by stroke. I am one of them, and from here on I have to live with serious disability. In my case the hereditary factor was not taken seriously. My Mother suffered from four mild strokes. When she was seventy- four she passed away from a sudden stroke. Her own Mother died at the age of fifty- one from a haemorrhagic stroke. I also suffer from high blood pressure, and was, therefore at risk of stroke. I had been taking medicaton for high blood pressure for at least twelve years before I suffered an acute stroke. Doctors in the hospital told me that the medication was no longer working for me. I, like my Grandmother, suffered a haemorrhagic stroke.

People can take precautions, by changing their lifestyles, to help prevent stroke. Regular exercise helps lower blood pressure. By keeping alcohol consumption down to one drink daily and by avoiding smoking altogether goes a long way towards stroke prevention. Medication prescribed for high blood pressure needs to be taken as prescribed, and must not be missed. If high blood pressure has been diagnosed the patient needs to have regular checks to make sure that the pressure is being kept well down. I purchased a wrist monitor, and I check my blood pressure from time to time. It's very reassuring to know that the pressure is at a safe level.